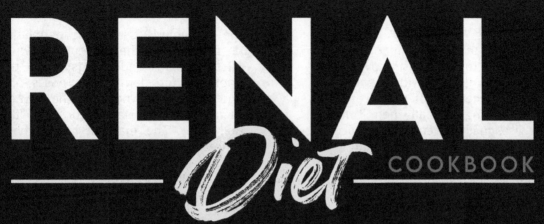

RENAL
Diet COOKBOOK

250 EASY AND DELICIOUS RECIPES WITH LOW QUANTITIES OF SODIUM, PHOSPHORUS, AND POTASSIUM FOR A PRACTICAL AND LOW BUDGET RENAL DIET

250
DELICIOUS RECIPES

AMOUNTS OF SODIUM, POTASSIUM, AND PHOSPHORUS INDICATED

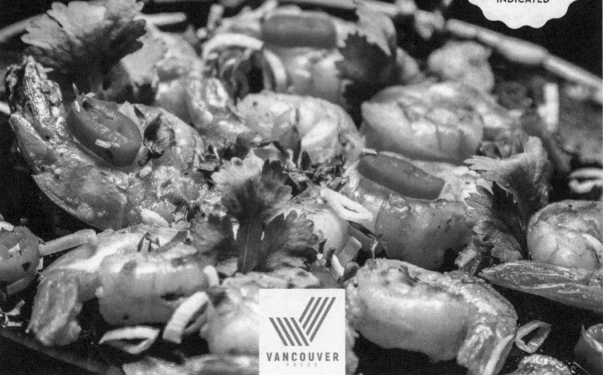

VANCOUVER
PRESS

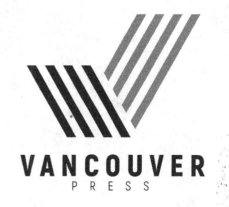

CONTENTS

INTRODUCTION 5

1. KIDNEY FRIENDLY DIET ON A
BUDGET 12

2. INGREDIENTS AND RECIPE
SUBSTITUTIONS GOOD FOR YOUR KIDNEY 20

3. GOING OUT TO EAT ON A KIDNEY DIET 28

4. THE 35 QUICKEST MEALS TO PREPARE 35

5. THE IMPORTANCE OF HERBS AND
SPICES IN YOUR DIET 39

6. FOOD LABELS AND HOW TO READ THEM 45

7. OVER 200 DELICIOUS RECIPES 48

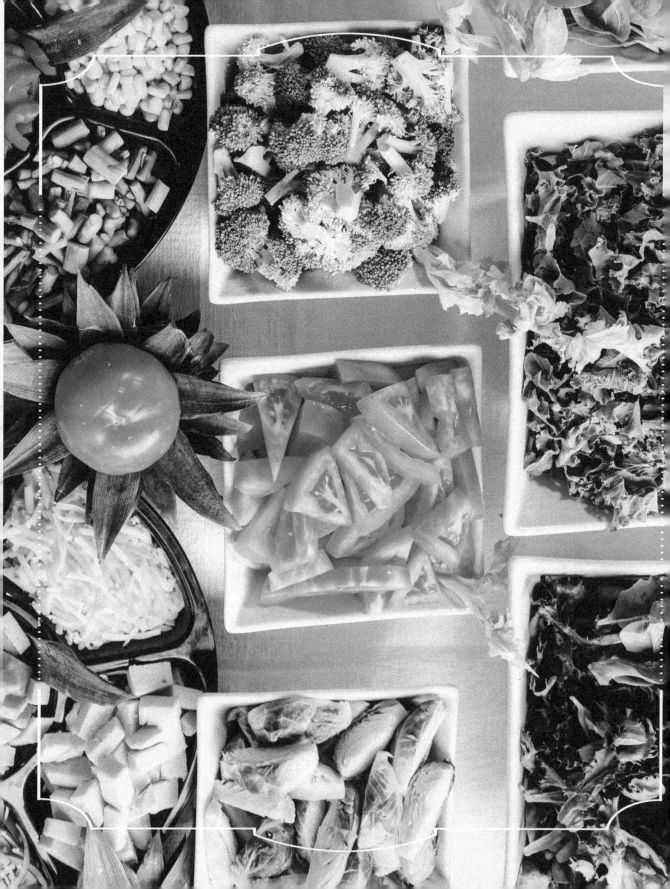

INTRODUCTION

This book was created with the intention of providing quick and practical recipes for those suffering from kidney dysfunction. We will not go into all the scientific elements of the disease, and we do not intend to replace your doctor's advice. Our intent is to provide the basic information on the recipes we propose clearly and simply. Each recipe provides the key nutritional values to fight kidney dysfunction, namely sodium, potassium, and phosphorus. This way, when combined with the instructions you will receive from your doctor, you can easily calculate the intake of these nutrients and choose the recipes that best suit your daily needs.

In the table at the beginning of the book, we found a quick and easy way to let you choose your favorite recipes. Next to the name of each meal are the total amounts of sodium, phosphorus, and potassium and the page number.
250 delicious, succulent, and healthy recipes are waiting to be prepared; good life!

Dish	DISHES	SOD.	POT.	PHOS.	
Sweet Potato Fries	Appetizers	8	132	18	50
Cream Cheese & Onion Dip	Appetizers	58	35	19	50
Cream Cheese & Pineapple	Appetizers	107	80	37	50
Pimento Cheese	Appetizers	107	80	37	50
Individual Frittatas	Appetizers	115	162	134	51
Spicy Pinwheels	Appetizers	162	63	38	51
Cream Cheese & Onion Dip	Appetizers	185	264	80	51
Crab Cakes With Lime Ginger Sauce	Appetizers	444	279	133	52
Sweet Potato Burrito	Appetizers	550	450	165	52
Louisiana BBQ Shrimp	Appetizers	666	423	244	53
Strawberry Sorbet	Beverages	1	79	12	53
Cranberry Punch	Beverages	8	153	16	54
Hot Spiced Apple Juice	Beverages	63	47	5	54
Biscuits with Master Mix	Biscuits	171	81	51	54
Yeast Dinner Rolls	Breads & Starches	5	31	32	54
Giblet Gravy	Breads & Starches	13	31	16	55
Herb Rice Casserole	Breads & Starches	19	74	29	55
Rice O'Brien	Breads & Starches	32	125	64	56
Old Fashioned Pancakes	Breads & Starches	58	57	64	56
Cornbread Dressing	Breads & Starches	75	88	62	56
High Protein Bread	Breads & Starches	77	101	108	57
Blueberry Baked Bread	Breads & Starches	92	83	20	58
White Bread Dressing	Breads & Starches	129	77	30	58
Blueberry Muffins	Breads & Starches	139	71	94	58
Baking Powder Biscuits	Breads & Starches	150	36	63	59
French Toast	Breads & Starches	194	128	61	59
Herb Bread	Breads & Starches	208	44	37	60
Homemade Pan Sausage	Breakfast	22	87	53	60
Maple Sausage	Breakfast	43	183	129	60
Pumpkin Spiced	Breakfast	141	82	41	61
Vegetable Omelet	Breakfast	145	122	195	61
Mexican Brunch Eggs	Breakfast	147	240	91	62
Loaded Veggie Eggs	Breakfast	195	605	254	62
Pancakes with Master Mix	Breakfast	302	260	175	63
Jellied Cranberry Sauce	Christmas	1	16	2	63
Gingerbread Cookies	Christmas	4	130	105	63
Roasted Turkey	Christmas	57	256	182	64
Coconut Marshmallow Salad	Christmas	64	185	74	64
Spiced Eggnog	Christmas	78	149	83	64
Garlic Mashed Potatoes	Christmas	103	205	65	66
Pumpkin Pie	Christmas	133	89	21	66
Lighter Christmas pudding	Christmas	150	626	-	67
Easy Shepherd's Pie	Christmas	312	605	296	68
Fried Apples	Desserts	1	153	10	68
Raspberry Pear Sorbet	Desserts	2,8	168	27	69
Blueberry Squares	Desserts	3	38	17	69

	DISHES	SOD.	POT.	PHOS.	
Scarlet's Frozen Fantasy	Desserts	3	109	129	70
Rhubarb Squares	Desserts	8	192	46	70
Jeweled Cookies	Desserts	9	29	16	71
Fruit Salad	Desserts	9	120	15	71
Lemon Crispies	Desserts	12	20	23	71
Fruit In The Clouds	Desserts	20	152	29	72
Cream Cheese Cookies	Desserts	31	15	14	72
Baked Egg Custard	Desserts	34	30	42	72
Spiced Pound Cake	Desserts	45	51	25	73
Spritz Cookies	Desserts	56	29	22	73
Fruit Crunch (Crumb Top Pie)	Desserts	62	68	37	74
Ribbon Cakes	Desserts	65	17	27	74
Chocolate- Orange Raisin Cookies	Desserts	66	139	52	75
Strawberries Brulee	Desserts	68	207	59	75
Cornbread Muffins	Desserts	79	89	67	75
Pineapple Pudding	Desserts	80	120	71	76
Easter Egg Wreath	Desserts	93	100	73	76
Pineapple Pound Cake	Desserts	93	67	47	77
Frozen Lemon Dessert	Desserts	97	69	33	78
Gingersnap Cookies	Desserts	117	57	11	87
Ice Cream Pumpkin Pie	Desserts	118	90	51	79
No-Bake Peanut Butter Balls	Desserts	120	106	65	79
Pumpkin Souffle	Desserts	120	387	112	80
Pineapple Upside-Down Cake	Desserts	123	76	26	80
Old Fashioned Pound Cake	Desserts	127	108	139	81
Cream Cheese Pound Cake	Desserts	133	29	16	81
Chocolate Pie Shell	Desserts	135	47	24	81
Lemon Chess Pie	Desserts	161	73	69	82
Apple and Cream Cheese Torte	Desserts	176	102	34	82
Whipped Cream Pound Cake	Desserts	192	120	24	83
Chocolate Mint Cake	Desserts	231	94	82	83
Sunny Angel Food Cake	Desserts	192	123	131	84
Chocolate Mocha Cheesecake	Desserts	280	67	52	84
Apple Filled Crepes	Desserts	356	160	103	85
Zucchini Prov	Dinner	38	988	131	86
Roasted Paprika-Laced Cauliflower	Dinner	43	429	62	86
Seasoned Pork Chops	Dinner	60	332	199	86
Oven Blasted Vegetables	Dinner	62	243	67	87
Italian Meatballs	Dinner	72	199	125	87
Crispy Oven Fried Chicken	Dinner	74	150	120	87
Crock Pot White Chicken Chili	Dinner	75	845	321	88
Fast Roast Chicken Lemon & Herbs	Dinner	77	222	188	88
Chili Rice With Beef	Dinner	78	427	233	89
Stuffed Zucchini	Dinner	86	578	109	89
Fruit Vinegar Chicken	Dinner	106	335	227	90
Grilled Lemon Chicken Kebabs	Dinner	119	404	238	90

	DISHES	SOD.	POT.	PHOS.	
Honey Herb Glazed Turkey	Dinner	119	526	357	91
Texas Hash	Dinner	134	427	177	91
Parslied Onions and Pinto Beans	Dinner	140	207	432	92
Herb Breaded Chicken	Dinner	180	444	249	92
Pancit Guisado	Dinner	194	391	183	93
Master Ground Beef Mix	Dinner	215	482	256	93
Texas-Style Chili	Dinner	218	490	168	94
Stir-fry Pepper Steak	Dinner	220	624	275	94
Paella	Dinner	257	330	201	95
Chicken Lasagna With White Sauce	Dinner	277	317	179	95
Rain City Stuffed Shells	Dinner	277	191	270	96
Quick Fettuccine	Dinner	285	216	121	97
Spicy Honey Mustard Chicken	Dinner	287	237	183	97
Taco Pockets	Dinner	367	397	194	98
Jammin' Jambalaya	Dinner	400	314	170	98
Puffy Chili Rellenos Casserole	Dinner	420	388	325	99
Tuna Loaf	Dinner	456	141	109	99
Chicken with Cornbread Stuffing	Dinner	478	414	204	99
Healthy Chicken Nuggets	Dinner	484	384	284	100
Slow Cooker Gumbo	Dinner	503	335	231	100
Shrimp Salad with Cucumber Mint	Dinner	226	357	320	101
Master Mix	Dough	271	298	189	101
Chicken 'N Rice	Lunch	76	283	218	102
Turkey Burgers	Lunch	98	266	62	102
Seafood Croquettes	Lunch	337	184	191	103
Tuna-Nood le Skillet Dinner	Lunch	407	515	228	103
Supreme of Seafood	Lunch	445	255	148	104
Speedy Tortilla Wraps	Lunch	233	156	89	104
Russian Tea	Lunch/Dinner	0	25	17	104
Gobi Curry	Lunch/Dinner	25	152	27	105
Swedish Meatballs	Lunch/Dinner	31	70	44	105
Fiesta Lime Fajitas	Lunch/Dinner	35	105	112	106
Stuffed Green Pepper	Lunch/Dinner	36	160	83	106
Confetti Chicken 'N Rice	Lunch/Dinner	37	316	152	107
Stir Fry Meal	Lunch/Dinner	37	618	26	107
Jalapeno Pepper Chicken	Lunch/Dinner	45	160	127	108
Kickin' Chicken Tacos	Lunch/Dinner	50	220	155	108
Orange-Glazed Chicken	Lunch/Dinner	56	353	182	108
Grilled Pork Souvlaki	Lunch/Dinner	58	336	179	109
Dilled fish	Lunch/Dinner	63	350	194	109
Crab Cakes	Lunch/Dinner	67	72	43	110
Fiesta Lime Tacos	Lunch/Dinner	70	140	111	110
Basic Meat Loaf	Lunch/Dinner	71	138	87	110
Cider Cream Chicken	Lunch/Dinner	83	414	266	111
Baked Fish	Lunch/Dinner	86	452	252	111
Curry Chicken	Lunch/Dinner	93	317	214	112

	DISHES	SOD.	POT.	PHOS.	
Chicken Stew	Lunch/Dinner	93	453	129	112
Parsley Burger	Lunch/Dinner	108	289	180	113
Oven Fried Chicken	Lunch/Dinner	109	234	172	113
New Orleans-Style Rice Dressing	Lunch/Dinner	113	377	228	113
Fajitas	Lunch/Dinner	121	494	207	114
Taco Stuffing	Lunch/Dinner	124	258	150	114
Salisbury Steak	Lunch/Dinner	128	366	218	115
Fish Tacos	Lunch/Dinner	138	335	181	115
Fast Fajitas	Lunch/Dinner	142	445	332	116
Spicy Lamb	Lunch/Dinner	144	423	237	116
One-Pot Chicken and Dumplings	Lunch/Dinner	146	455	227	116
Crunchy Chicken Nuggets	Lunch/Dinner	176	237	134	117
Rosemary, Lemon, and Mustard	Lunch/Dinner	180	46	2	118
Turkey & Noodles	Lunch/Dinner	188	533	296	118
Strip Steak With Smothered Onions	Lunch/Dinner	200	360	200	118
Beef or Chicken Enchiladas	Lunch/Dinner	201	222	146	119
Pasta Without tomato sauce	Lunch/Dinner	227	269	89	119
Mediterranean Lamb Patties	Lunch/Dinner	229	45	74	120
Fish Sticks	Lunch/Dinner	240	224	130	120
Open-Faced Steak & Onion Sandwich	Lunch/Dinner	247	200	115	121
Rotini with Mock Italian Sausage	Lunch/Dinner	250	458	161	121
Dijon Chicken	Lunch/Dinner	258	454	250	122
Eggplant Casserole	Lunch/Dinner	263	380	169	122
Chicken Seafood Gumbo	Lunch/Dinner	320	426	156	123
Pasta with Pesto	Lunch/Dinner	336	476	237	123
Barbecue Cups	Lunch/Dinner	342	151	152	124
Creamy Tuna Twist	Lunch/Dinner	379	204	122	124
Broccoli Chicken Casserole	Lunch/Dinner	388	371	243	124
Alaska Baked Macaroni and Cheese	Lunch/Dinner	479	237	428	125
Turkey Paprikash	Lunch/Dinner	484	481	356	125
Special Pizza	Pizzas	144	188	31	126
Beef and Bell Pepper Pizza	Pizzas	150	352	230	127
Dessert Pizza	Pizzas	166	98	47	127
Mediterranean Pizza	Pizzas	240	86	90	128
English Muffin Pizza	Pizzas	529	324	254	128
BBQ Rub For Pork or Chicken	Rubs	9	34	7	128
Fire and Ice Watermelon Salsa	Salads	2	128	14	129
Tabbouleh	Salads	7	180	66	129
Italian Dressing	Salads	18	10	1	129
Green Garden Salad	Salads	20	215	29	130
Berry Wild Rice Salad	Salads	21	214	98	130
Raspberry Vinaigrette	Salads	21	14	2	131
Lemon Curry Chicken Salad	Salads	46	221	82	131
Sunshine Salad	Salads	64	119	25	131
Thai Salad with Corn	Salads	84	162	15	132
Pasta Salad with Roasted Red Sauce	Salads	85	150	91	132

	DISHES	SOD.	POT.	PHOS.	
Chicken N' Orange Salad Sandwich	Salads	93	241	106	133
Macaroni Salads	Salads	103	106	74	133
Potato Salad	Salads	206	174	45	133
Apple Rice Salad	Salads	227	238	82	134
Shrimp Salad	Salads	232	233	263	134
Chicken Salad Delight	Salads	239	205	149	135
Chicken Vegetable Salad	Salads	245	230	143	135
Salt-Free Sweet Brown Mustard	Sauces	2	27	18	135
Low Salt Guacamole	Sauces	4	89	3	136
Relish	Sauces	8	31	9	136
Sour Cream Dill Sauce	Sauces	15	48	25	136
Low Salt Ketchup	Sauces	17	62	1	136
Simple White Sauce	Sauces	25	54	43	137
Spicy Barbecue Sauce	Sauces	28	34	7	137
Homemade Low-Sodium Soy Sauce	Sauces	38	113	3	138
Alfredo Sauce	Sauces	142	32	75	138
Pico de gallo	Sauces	294	144	19	139
Steamed Asparagus	Side Dishes	1	123	32	139
Roasted Green Beans and Sweet Onion	Side Dishes	6	161	15	139
Wild Rice Stuffing	Side Dishes	10	611	146	140
Fried Onion Rings	Side Dishes	11	99	39	140
Hearty Mashed Potatoes	Side Dishes	13	180	61	140
Marinated Vegetables	Side Dishes	13	154	39	141
Green Beans with Hazelnuts	Side Dishes	19	246	73	141
Fragrant & Flavorful Basmati Rice	Side Dishes	25	49	17	142
Vegetables & Rice	Side Dishes	32	99	67	142
Kale and Turnip Greens	Side Dishes	33	335	45	143
Baked Yellow Squash	Side Dishes	34	139	25	143
Honey Glazed Carrots	Side Dishes	75	256	39	143
Almost Mashed Potatoes	Side Dishes	76	198	54	144
Favorite Green Beans	Side Dishes	77	214	38	144
Purple and Gold Thai Coleslaw	Side Dishes	79	228	29	144
Pineapple Coleslaw	Side Dishes	81	143	14	145
Coleslaw	Side Dishes	81	76	14	145
Pulled Pork BBQ style	Side Dishes	90	652	241	145
Summer Salad	Side Dishes	95	265	104	146
Beef Jerky	Side Dishes	100	100	190	146
Fruit Omelet	Side Dishes	125	430	141	147
Herbed Omelet	Side Dishes	157	157	214	147
Coleslaw with a Kick	Side Dishes	170	117	11	148
Yellow Squash & Green Onions	Side Dishes	347	204	40	148
Brown Bag Popcorn	Snacks	0	105	96	148
Pita Wedges	Snacks	161	30	45	149
Chicken Nood le Soup	Soups	17	101	39	149
Beef & Vegetable Soup	Soups	56	291	121	150
Simple Chicken Broth	Soups	67	196	55	150

DISHES	SOD.	POT.	PHOS.	
Beef Barley Soup	Soups	105	678	250	150
Baked Potato Soup	Soups	272	594	326	151
Thai Chicken Soup	Soups	300	800	382	151

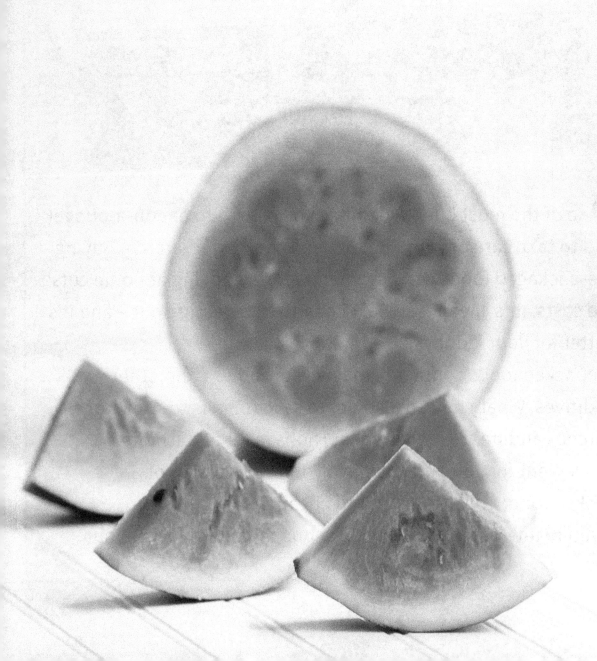

1

KIDNEY FRIENDLY DIET ON A BUDGET

One of the most effective things you can do to eat on-a-budget and to take care of your kidneys is to cook from scratch. Buying pre-packaged foods can be expensive, so, cooking at home cuts the costs. It is cheap – at least cheaper than eating out – and it's better for your kidneys.

Prepacked foods contain high levels of sodium and other additives. What you can also do, to save time, is to cook large batches and freeze individual portions, so that it's more convenient for you and you have your own version of pre-packed food; only healthier and cheaper.

If you're interested in eating on-a-budget and reducing your grocery bill, check out the tips down below.

Vegetable and Fruit

- **Buy products that are in season**, it will be less expensive because you're not paying the landed cost of the imported products and they will also taste better.

  Winter – turnips, onions, carrots, potatoes.
  Spring – strawberries, rhubarb, lettuce.
  Summer – cherries, berries, peaches, corn, green/yellow beans, cucumbers.
  Fall – apples, pears, plums, grapes, cabbage, broccoli, cauliflower.

- **Added sauces**, seasonings and sugars are to be avoided. Make sure your frozen vegetables and your fruit contain any. Buy fresh products if can and are not concerned about the spoiling date. Products without anything added to them are less expensive and you get to choose the exact amount of sauces, seasonings and sugars you want to add.

- **Purchase canned vegetables or fruit** with the label "no salt added" and "no sugar added". Canned products are less expensive, but they tend to have a lot of sodium and/or sugar added.

- **Purchase fresh fruit and vegetables** at different stage of ripeness, so that you know which one to eat first and which one can wait a few days before it spoils.

Non-expansive purchases:

- Cabbage, carrots, potatoes, turnips, onions, apples.
- Fresh products in season.
- Canned tomatoes (look out for those with no added salt).

Non-expansive purchases:

- Skim milk powder.
- Plain yogurt.

Grain products

- To maintain your bread fresh, wrap it well and put it in the freezer. Remove slices when you need it.

- Stock up when pasta is on sale; it can last several years if unopened and kept in the dark.

- Buy plain cereals rather that those sweetened varieties. Add fruit for sweetness if desired.

Non-expansive purchases:

- Parboiled rice.
- Macaroni, spaghetti, noodles.
- Hot cereals, plain ready-to-eat cereals.

Meat and Alternatives

- Eggs are a great source of proteins and they're also cheap.
- Peanut butter is also a cheap source of proteins, but should be limited to one serving per day.
- Buy canned light tuna and pink salmon; it's less expensive. Make sure to rinse thoroughly to remove sodium.
- It's cheaper to buy larger cuts of meat, so, instead of buying chicken breasts, buy a whole chicken. Divide in in individual portions and freeze it, or cook the entire chicken and freeze later. You can reheat it and it's a ready-to-eat meal. You can also

share some with friends.

- If you're freezer is large, buy meat when it's on sale. Divide the meat into individual portions and before freezing it, write the date on it.
- Try having a meatless meal once or twice a week. There are many alternatives, such as scrambled eggs, omelets or tofu.

Non-expansive purchases:

- Less tender meat such as blade, chuck, flank, round, stewing meat, ground beef.
- Whole poultry, grade B or utility grade, chicken legs.
- Eggs.
- Beans, lentils, peanut butter.
- Pork butt, loin or rib, pork chops.
- Canned fish (look for low sodium varieties).

Other Foods

Avoid buying high-energy or low nutrients foods, such as soft drinks, chocolate, chips and other unhealthy snacks. They're not only expensive, they also don't have any essential vitamin or minerals needed for a healthy diet.

Shopping at the Grocery Store

- It recommended that you check the grocery store flyers and plan your meals around what's on sale and most importantly, choose the products healthier for your kidneys.
- Plan your meals ahead of time, write a grocery list and stick to it. Avoid buying on an impulse.
- Compare costs among different grocery stores and find the cheapest options.
- Compare prices between name brands and generic brands.
- Find coupons in the newspaper flyers, internet or at the store and use them for the products you need. As long as you're saving money and the name brand costs less than the generic brand with the coupon.
- It is less expansive to buy club pack items and if you don't think you'll be able to use it all, share it with friends and family.
- Try buying lower grade meat and produce. Grade A and grade B have the same nutrients, grade A only has a better appearance.
- Bring your own bags to avoid buying some at the grocery store.

Check out these alternative places to buy fresh products, take along a list of low and high potassium foods if you need to restrict potassium:

- Farmer's Markets
- Farm Gate Stands
- Community Gardens
- Community Shared Agriculture
- Good Food Box Programs

Other Foods

- Self---Help Food Banks (Allow you to choose your own items to tailor to your kidney diet).
- Community Meals or Hamper Programs (Often run through local churches or community programs).

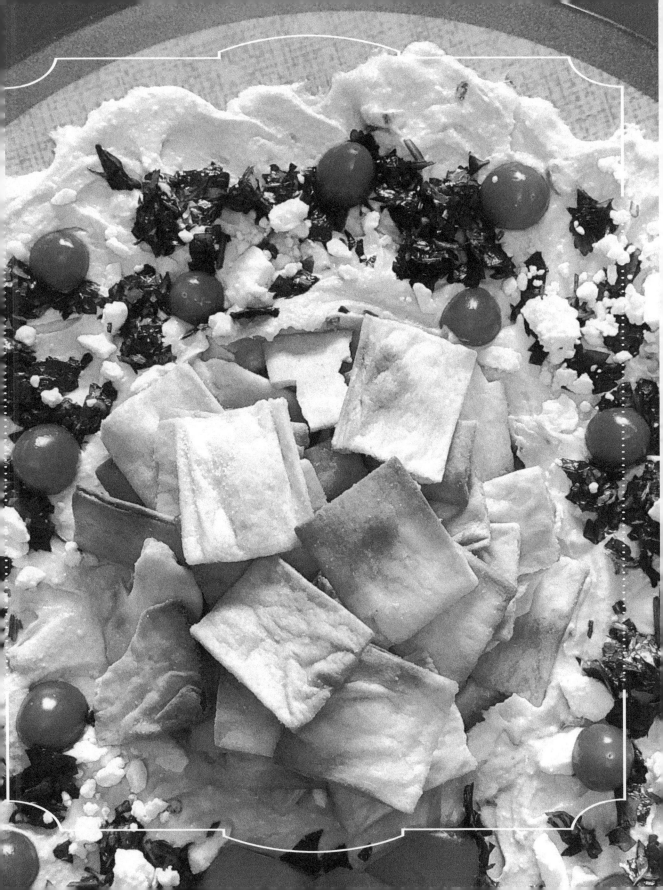

2

INGREDIENTS AND RECIPE SUBSTITUTIONS GOOD FOR YOUR KIDNEY

Baking and cooking from scratch on a kidney-friendly diet can be challenging. It is not impossible though; with the right products and substitutions you can cook your favorite meals!

It is best that you cook your food, because the already pre-made products you see at the store are high in sodium, potassium, phosphorus and calcium.

You might have to make some changes to make sure you're meeting all your nutrient needs and are following your dietary plan.

Baking Ingredients and Kidney Friendly Substitutions

Some ingredients can't be removed from a recipe to make it taste the way it does, so tweaking the ingredients that will act as a substitute to ensure the right mixture if fat, liquids and leavening agents is important.

Leavening agents are often used in foods like cakes and pastries to help them rise and, they can often contain high levels of phosphorus, potassium and sodium. Another ingredient high in sodium and phosphorus is baking powder, but low sodium baking powder is high in potassium, so be careful when choosing baking powder for your recipes. Check the nutrition facts table to see how much sodium, phosphorus and potassium the product contains. The same way baking soda can be a large source of sodium, Cream of tartar can be a large source of potassium. Again, check the nutrition facts table to find products low in sodium and potassium. Other kidney friendly substitutions for recipe ingredients are:

Kidney Friendly Substitutions

Baking Ingredient	Problem Nutrients	Kidney Friendly Substitution
Whole wheat flour	High in potassium and phosphorus	Any white flour
Self---rising flour	High in sodium and phosphorus	All-purpose white flour
Regular butter or margarine	High in sodium	Unsalted butter or non---hydrogenated margarine
Sugar (for diabetics)	Adds additional carbohydrate	Sugar substitutes
Eggs	Higher in cholesterol and phosphorus	Egg whites or egg substitutes
Salt	High in sodium	Reduce amount of salt in recipes. Alternatively, herbs and spices can be used – nutmeg, cinnamon, low sodium spices
Milk	High in potassium and phosphorus	Unenriched almond or rice beverage (any flavor except chocolate)

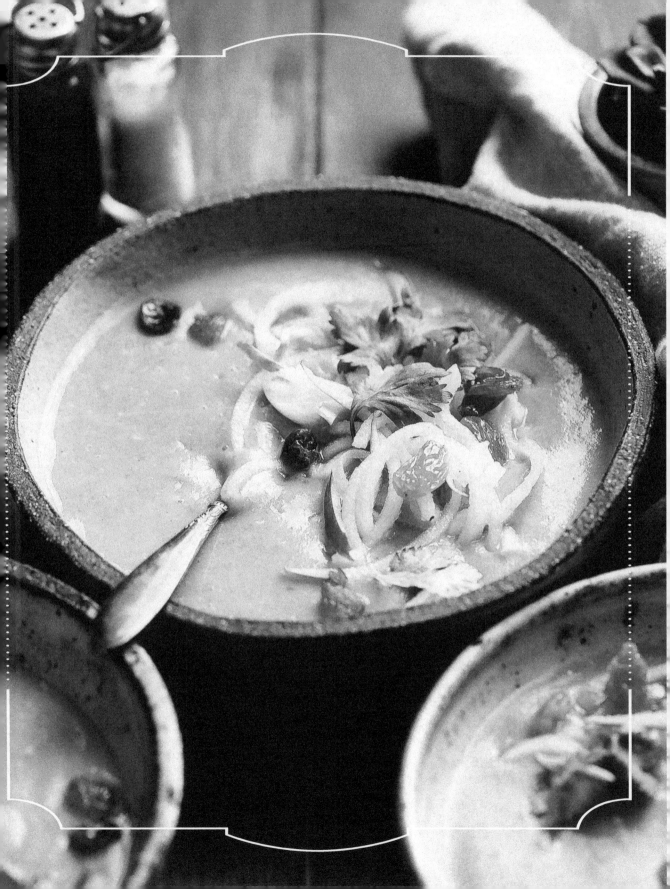

If you decide to buy baked goods

If you're purchasing pastries from the bakery, making substitutions won't be possible.

Avoid buying items with the following ingredients:

- Chocolate or cocoa (powder)
- Items containing banana
- Items containing nuts or peanut butter
- Items containing large amounts of milk (including condensed and evaporated milk)

Kidney friendly baked items to eat in moderation

- Sugar cookies or spice cookies
- Shortbread
- Vanilla wafers
- Vanilla/white cake
- Angel food cake
- Lemon flavored cakes and pastries
- Apple, berry and peach pie
- Breads: sourdough, white, French, Italian
- Cinnamon rolls

- Bagels (avoid whole wheat and bagels containing raisins) – blueberry, plain, sesame

Any recipe can be adapted to be more kidney friendly, down below some suggestions to make your favorite recipes with little potassium, sodium, phosphorus and calcium.

If you're trying to lower your phosphorus intake, consider making these changes:

- Substitute milk with unenriched rice or almond beverage, but make sure it's not chocolate flavored.
- Use small amounts of cheese when called for in a recipe, or choose cream cheese if it's better for the recipe you're making.
- If possible, omit nuts from the recipe.
- Try using a small amount of whipped topping, if whipping cream is called for in a dessert.
- Use fresh meat choices – baked, barbecued, roasted or broiled – in place of processed meats.

These suggestions will help you reduce your sodium intake as well.
If you're trying to lower your potassium intake, consider making

these changes:

- Peel, cut and boil potatoes, carrots and broccoli in a separate pot of water to leach potassium before draining and adding to the soup or stew.
- Avoid tomato sauces – try a small amount of fresh tomato instead, or if you're cooking pasta, use small amounts of olive oil and garlic in place of the tomato sauce. This is a good substitute for cream sauces which are high in phosphorus.
- Choose low potassium fruits and vegetables whenever possible.
- Try choosing pasta or white rice instead of potatoes. Mashed cauliflower is a good alternative to mashed potatoes.

If you're trying to lower your sodium intake, consider making these changes:

- Make your own low sodium salad dressings, oil and balsamic vinegar are a sodium free choice.
- If using nuts in a recipe, choose the unsalted variety.
- Choose low sodium canned foods whenever possible. Rinsing canned vegetables and legumes such as kidney beans and chickpeas can help reduce the sodium content.
- Add a variety of herbs and seasonings to flavor your foods.

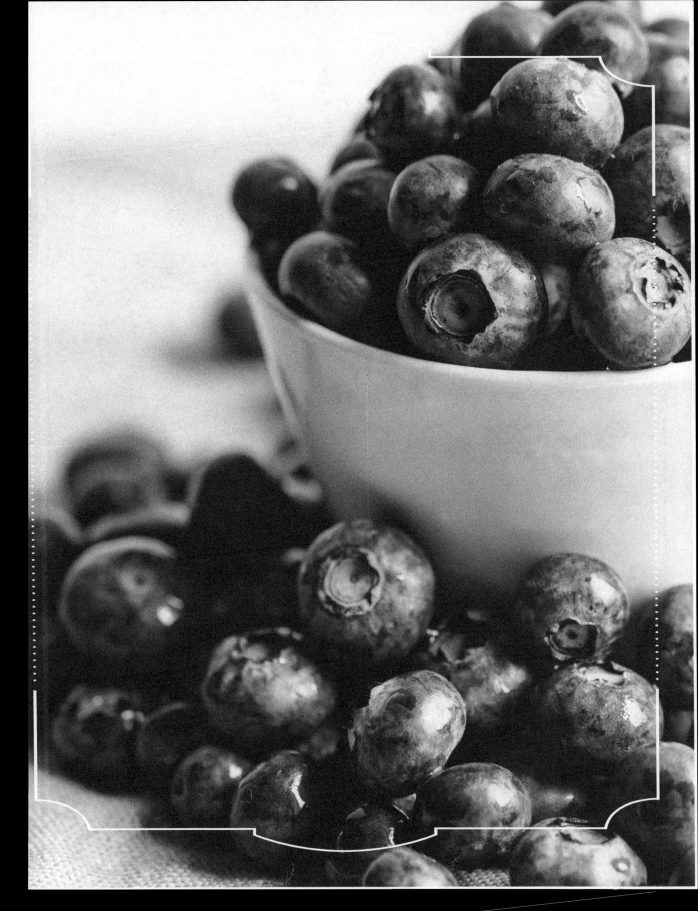

3

GOING OUT TO EAT ON A KIDNEY DIET

Going out to eat is a social outing and a break from cooking, but following a dietary plan when eating out at a restaurant can be a challenge, but it can be managed. Nowadays, a lot of restaurants post their menus online; you can plan your options ahead by looking at their online menu and if there's nothing kidney friendly, you can call them and ask them to prepare something specific for you.

Plan Ahead

- Review your kidney diet before you go out or bring your food lists with you.
- If you know you will be eating out, eat less throughout the day and avoid any salty or high potassium foods.
- If you're on a fluid restriction, save your fluids throughout the day so that you can have more when eating out.
- If you're on phosphate binders, remember to bring them with you when you're out eating.

Read the menu carefully

- Ask questions about any menu items you are not sure about. Servers are used to being asked questions about the items on the menu.
- If you're not comfortable asking questions in front of your friends, call ahead the restaurant and check the menu online. Many restaurants have nutritional information available.

Special requests

- Many restaurants are not willing to make big changes in their meals, for instance, they are happy to make substitutions in the choice of salad dressing, sauces and gravies, or rice instead of potatoes, but not big changes.

- Ask them if your meal can be cooked without extra or added salt. Explain why you'd rather avoid big amounts of salt and make sure they understand your request is important. Calling ahead is better than waiting until the last minute.

Everything that you'll order at a restaurant will be saltier than what you have at home, moderation is key.

Menu choices

Appetizers and Salads

- Share with friends.
- Look for fresh items and avoid a heavy salt or fluid load.
- Ask which fruits and vegetables are in the salad if it's not specified in the menu.
- Avoid ordering a salad if it contains bacon, ham, nuts or croutons.
- Ask for oil and vinegar salad dressing to avoid the extra salt in prepared dressings.

- Better choices: Green salad, crab cakes, shrimps, cocktail garlic bread without cheese, fried zucchini or onion rings.

Entrees

- Watch your portion sizes and try to eat the same way you would eat at home. If it's too much ask for a container to take the extra at home.
- Avoid mixing dishes which are often higher in salt and phosphorus.
- Avoid cream sauces, gravies and soy sauce.
- Remove the skin from poultry to help decrease the salt content.
- Season food with fresh ground pepper, lemon or lime juice to add flavor instead of using salt.
- Better choices: grilled or broiled steaks, lamb chops, prime rib, hamburger without cheese, fajitas, chicken (fried, grilled or roasted), sandwiches.

Side Dishes

- Choose starches and vegetables lower in potassium if you're on a potassium restriction.
- Save your fruit and vegetables choices during the day if you

know you will be eating out.

- Ask for a substitute if necessary.
- Better choices: rice, noodles, green beans, mixed vegetables.

Desserts

- Ask for a clear description of the dessert
- Avoid chocolate, cream cheese, ice cream or nuts which will be higher in potassium and phosphorus.
- Low potassium fruits make a good dessert choice, especially if you have diabetes.
- Share your dessert with your friends.
- Better choices: low potassium fruit, fruit ice, sorbet, apple, blueberry, lemon meringue pies, strawberry shortcake.

Beverages

- If your diet requires a fluid restriction, ask for a small glass and drink slowly. Even if it's water.
- Decline drink refills so that you can monitor your fluid intake.
- Avoid beer, colas, tomato or clam juice.
- Choose clear pops, sparkling water and juices found on your meal plan.

When eating out make sure you take your time to enjoy your food, be grateful for the company and remember that eating out is a necessity and not a pleasure. Plan ahead and play it safe.

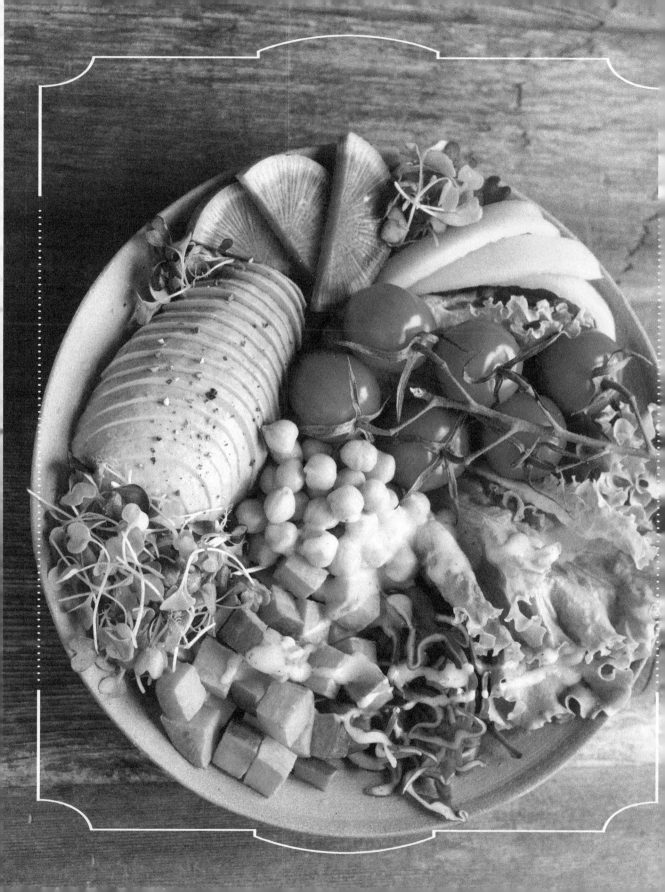

4

THE 35 QUICKEST MEALS TO PREPARE

Cheese and Onion Omelet, a salad:

1. French toast & berries
2. Grilled Cheese sandwich, celery & pepper strips with dip
3. Shish Kebabs (beef/lamb cubes, green/red pepper, onion on skewer) & rice
4. Spaghetti (noodles with meat sauce), salad
5. Breakfast sandwich: egg, cheese on an English muffin
6. Hamburger, macaroni salad, watermelon
7. Unsalted crackers with tuna, chicken or egg salad

8. Meatloaf, mashed potatoes, frozen vegetables

9. Peanut butter and pear on bread

10. English muffin with cheese melted under broiler

11. Tuna melt (Split English muffin halves, top with tuna, mayonnaise and cheese, broil)

12. Egg salad with sprouts on cracked wheat bread

13. Cottage cheese, fruit salad, zucchini loaf

14. Hard cooked egg, coleslaw, buttered bread

15. Chicken or turkey, slice of tomato, lettuce on Kaiser

16. Tuna casserole, salad, fruit

17. Homemade macaroni and cheese, broccoli or cauliflower

18. Salad plate: sliced turkey, hard-boiled egg, lettuce, cottage cheese, crackers

19. Low sodium soup (try "Soup's On" for a readymade low salt soup), crackers with Brie cheese

20. Spread peanut butter over pita bread. Slice fresh apples over top, sprinkle with cinnamon, and broil for 3 to 5 minutes.

21. Chicken on light rye, raw veggies, fruit cocktail

22. Top flour tortillas with diced tomatoes and green pepper, diced leftover chicken, and grated cheese. Fold in half, and bake in the oven until heated through. Cut into wedges, and serve with salsa and sour cream

23. Peanut butter, crackers, apple

24. Salad topped with tuna or cottage cheese, bread with margarine, fruit

25. Meatballs, rice, peas, fruit cocktail

26. Broiled fish, couscous, salad with mandarins

27. Tuna pasta salad, applesauce

28. Stir fry chicken & vegetables, rice

29. Chicken on pita with cucumbers & lettuce, salad dressing

30. Roast beef sandwich, raw veggies

31. Turkey on bagel, cucumber salad, juice

32. Salmon sandwich, green salad, peach

33. Chicken breast, green beans, roll

34. Mini pizzas — Spoon pizza sauce onto half a bagel, English muffin, or mini pita. Top with mozzarella cheese, cooked chicken and your favorite veggies, bake at a low setting until the cheese is melted and the bagel is crispy.

35. Mix leftover chicken with sliced grapes, mayonnaise, dash of curry powder. Stuff into pita pocket.

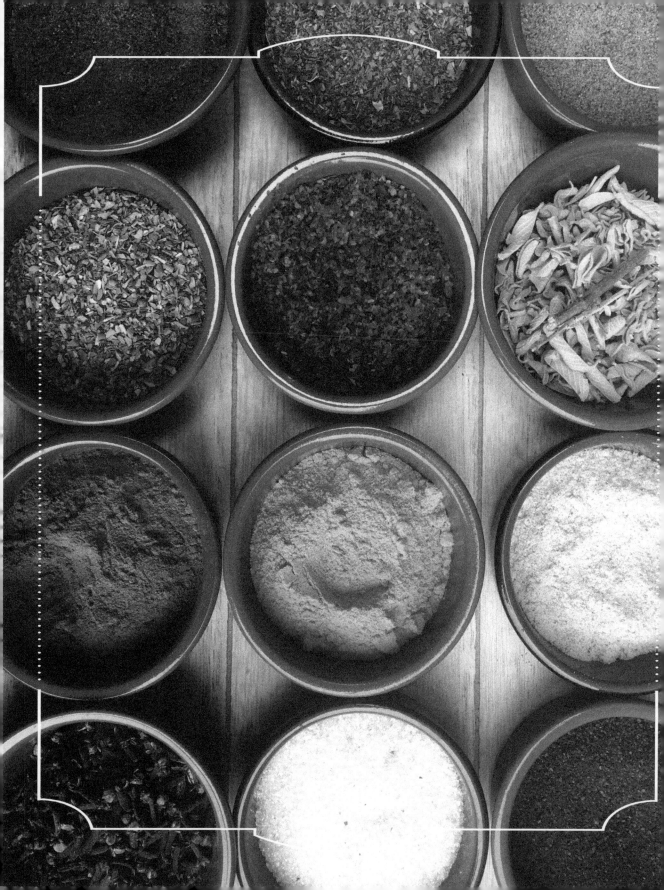

5

THE IMPORTANCE OF HERBS AND SPICES IN YOUR DIET

Spice and herbs not only improve the taste of your food, but they also have health benefits. Research shows potential benefits of spices and herbs, rich in antioxidants and excellent sources of other vitamins and minerals.

Science is currently examining the compounds that make up these herbs and spices, and more than 2,000 have been identified in herbs and spices. They might even contain lower levels if compared

Cutting out sugar, salt and fat is easier when you have a flavorful replacement that is also kidney friendly. You can start with your new diet right away, because these herbs and spices are easy to incorporate into everyday meals.

Here are seven kidney friendly seasonings to spice up your diet:

ROSEMARY

This herb is found to be important for your brain health, memory and cognition. Before baking frozen dinner-rolls brush them with some olive oil and sprinkle the rolls with some crushed rosemary leaves. You can also add it to chicken or vegetable soup, and maybe even adding oregano and thyme.

GARLIC

Garlic has antibacterial and antioxidants benefits. To give more flavor to your meals, add garlic powder or crushed garlic to pasta, rice or cooked vegetables. You can also make your version of garlic bread, by mixing olive oil with fresh garlic or garlic powder and brushing it over the slice of bread. Broil it for 2-3 minutes.

OREGANO

This herb is high in vitamin K, important for bone and blood health. Sprinkle oregano on your garlic bread to have that traditional "pizza taste" without adding extra tomato sauce and potassium. You can also mix oregano and garlic powder and add this mix to your pasta.

CHILI

Chili peppers are a good source of vitamin A, important for the eye and skin health. Studies shows that consuming chili peppers might boost your metabolism. If you're not a fan of spicy foods, you can always incorporate this spice in meals without burning your tongue. There's a spicy spectrum and you can choose the least spicy.

From the most to the least spicy: cayenne, crushed red pepper, black pepper, paprika.

These spices are easy to add to your diet by sprinkling them over your meals. You can for example, sprinkle some paprika to your eggs, tuna or chicken salad or add cayenne pepper to your favorite vinaigrette. An excess of vitamin A is to be avoided to those with kidney failure.

GINGER

It's a root known to aid digestion and help with nausea. It has many inflammatory, antioxidants and pain relief properties that are a great addition to your diet. Ginger is often found in Asian recipes and it is easy to add to poultry and fish marinades. You can also add it to fruit salads and it complements green tea and lemonade.

CINNAMON

Recent researches show that this spice help regulate blood. It can be added to applesauce, cream of wheat or sliced raw or baked apples for a delicious and healthy snack.

BASIL

Basil adds flavor without adding high amounts of potassium or phosphorus. This herb can be included in everyday meals because it's easy to use. Try basil leaves instead of lettuce in your sandwich and use it as a garnish.

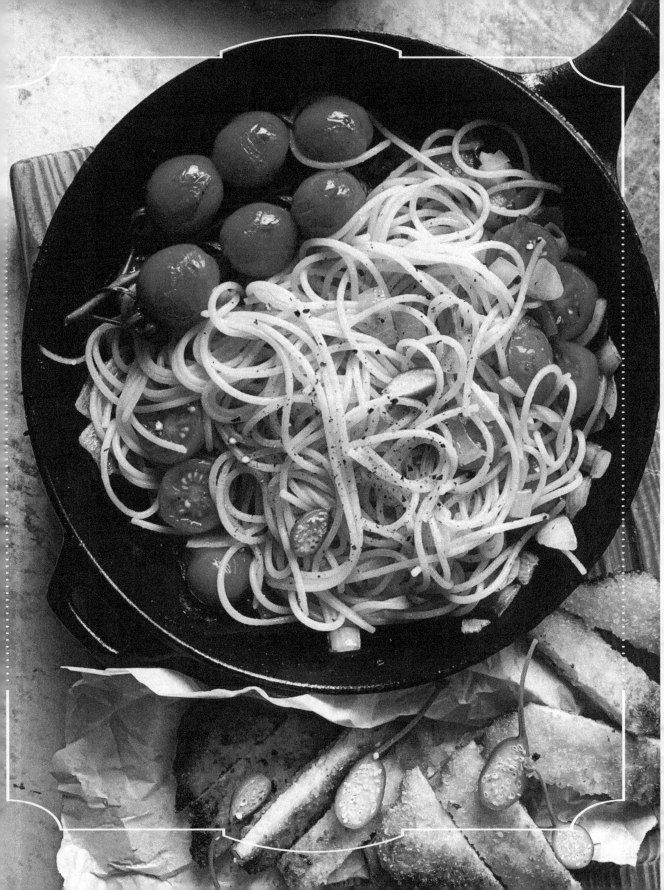

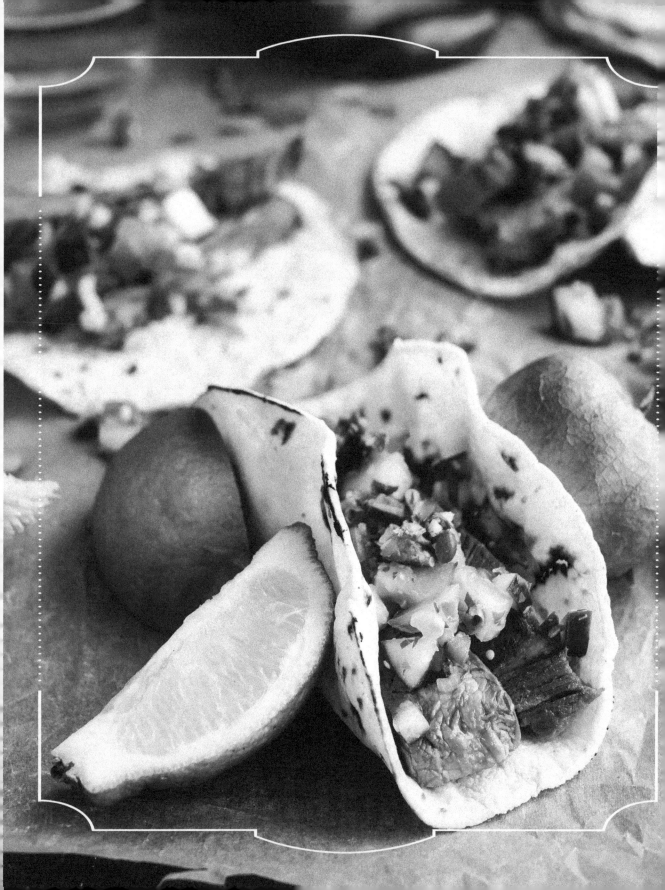

6

FOOD LABELS AND HOW TO READ THEM

Food labels are the tool that allows you to choose healthier and more kidney friendly foods.

Talk with your renal dietitian before you go grocery shopping as you will need to be aware of certain nutrients such as potassium and phosphorus. They can tell you how many milligrams or how much you should have each day. Once you know the right amount, you can start shopping. a gallon a day. This includes water in the beverages you drink, as well as the water contained in foods that you eat. Buy a BPA-free reusable water bottle and keep it with you so you can stay hydrated all day long.

Nutrition Facts		
8 servings per container		
Serving size		2/3 cup (55g)

Amount per 2/3 cup	
Calories	**230**

% DV*		
12%	**Total Fat** 8g	
5%	Saturated Fat 1g	
	Trans Fat 0g	
0%	**Cholesterol** 0mg	
7%	**Sodium** 160mg	
12%	**Total Carbs** 37g	
14%	Dietary Fiber 4g	
	Sugars 1g	
	Added Sugars 0g	
	Protein 3g	
10%	Vitamin D 2mcg	
20%	Calcium 260mg	
45%	Iron 8mg	
5%	Potassium 235mg	

* Footnote on Daily Values (DV) and calories reference to be inserted here.

General tips – The items you should look out are generally listed by content in grams or milligrams and percent daily values. These values are for people without a kidney disease, so your needs may differ.

Phosphorus – The rules says that good foods have less than 50 mg of phosphorus or less than 5%. If it has 150 mg or 15% or more of phosphorus you should avoid it.

Potassium – Good foods contain less than 100 mg or 3% of potassium. More than 200 mg or 6% is high.

Hidden minerals – Be careful, just because some minerals are not listed, it does not mean that they're not there.

Serving size – Another thing to look at is the serving size, a bottle of 20oz of soda has 2.5 servings for bottle. Drink the entire bottle and the values are multiplied by 2.5.

the values are multiplied by 2.5.

Readability – Carry around a small magnifying glass with you to read some labels because some prints are small and difficult to read.

Consult a Dietitian – If in doubt, save the labels and bring them with you to the next appointment with your dietician.

7

OVER 200 DELICIOUS RECIPES

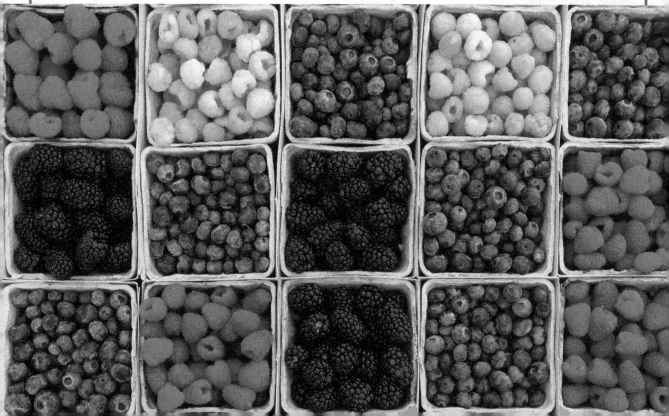

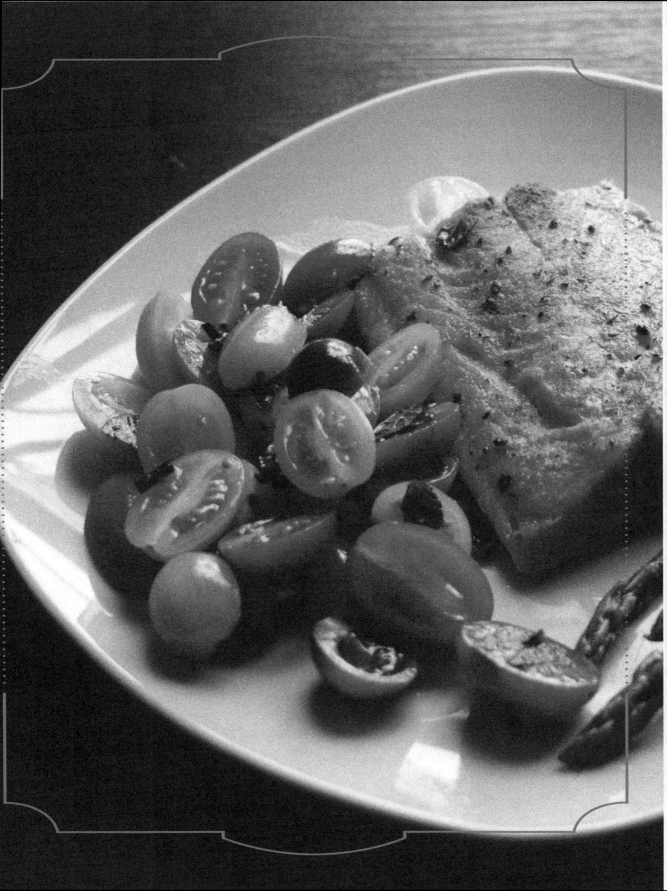

SWEET POTATO FRIES

Ingredients:
Based on 4 servings per recipe
2 sweet potatoes
small amount non-stick cooking spray or salad oil
Directions:
1. Preheat oven to 500 degrees.
2. Peel and slice sweet potatoes into 1/8" thick slices (soak to lower the potassium).
3. Spray cookie sheet with non-stick cooking spray or wipe with salad oil.
4. Place on a baking sheet, bake for 15 minute.

Nutrition Facts (per serving)
Calories 68 Carbohydrates 15 g
Protein 1 g Dietary Fiber 0 g
Fat 2 g Sodium 8 mg
Potassium 132 mg Phosphorus 18 mg

CREAM CHEESE & ONION DIP

Ingredients:
Yield: 20 servings Serving size: 1 teaspoon
¼ cup onion grated
8 ounces low-fat cream cheese, softened
1 teaspoon Tabasco® sauce
1 teaspoon onion powder
½ teaspoon black pepper 1 teaspoon chives
Directions:
1. Combine all ingredients and mix well
2. Serve with raw vegetables and/or unsalted crackers.

Nutrition Facts (per serving)
Calories 26 Carbohydrates 7 g

Protein 1 g Dietary Fiber 0 g
Fat 2 g Sodium 58 mg
Potassium 35 mg Phosphorus 19 mg

CREAM CHEESE & PINEAPPLE

Ingredients:
Yield: 7 servings Serving size: 2 tablespoons
1 cup crushed pineapple, drained well
1 8-ounce package cream cheese, softened
Directions:
Combine both ingredients in a mixing bowl

Nutrition Facts (per serving)
Calories 130 Carbohydrates 6 g
Protein 2 g Dietary Fiber 0 g
Fat 2 g Sodium 8 mg Potassium 80 mg
Phosphorus 37 mg

PIMENTO CHEESE

Ingredients:
Yield: 5 servings Serving size: 2 tablespoons
1 cup low sodium cheese, grated
¼ cup pimentos
2 tablespoons mayonnaise
Directions:
Combine all ingredients, mix well.

Nutrition Facts (per serving)
Calories 133 Carbohydrates 6 g
Protein 6 g Dietary Fiber 0 g
Fat 11 g Sodium 107 mg Potassium 80 mg Phosphorus 37 mg

INDIVIDUAL FRITTATAS

Ingredients:
Yield: 8 servings Serving size: 1 frittata
1 pound frozen hash brown potatoes
1/8 teaspoon black pepper
2 ounces cooked lean ham
2 tablespoons red bell pepper
2 tablespoons green bell pepper
2 tablespoons onion
4 large eggs
1 tablespoon 1% low-fat milk
1/2 cup shredded low-fat cheddar cheese

Directions:
1. Soak hash brown potatoes in a large bowl of water for 4 hours. Drain, rinse and squeeze out excess water. (Skip this step if low potassium is not needed.)
2. Preheat the oven to 375° F. Coat 8 muffin tin holes with cooking spray.
3. Using a 1/3 cup measure, place hash browns in muffin cups and press potato in the bottom and up the sides of each muffin cup. Spray the hash browns with cooking spray. Place in the oven and cook for 15 minutes and remove from oven. Reduce oven temperature to 350° F.
4. Finely chop the ham, peppers and onion. Beat the eggs and milk together in a medium bowl; season with black pepper. Add the ham, peppers, onion and cheese to egg mixture and combine.
5. Press partially baked hash browns down firmly with a spoon so that potatoes cover the bottom and sides of each muffin hole. Pour 1/4-cup egg mixture into the center of each muffin hole.
6. Return the pan to the oven and cook until potatoes are crisp and golden and

Nutrition Facts (per serving)
Calories 112 Carbohydrates 11 g
Protein 8 g Dietary Fiber 1 g
Fat 4 g Sodium 115 mg
Potassium 162 mg Phosphorus 134 mg

SPICY PINWHEELS

Ingredients:
Yield: 120 Pinwheels Serving size: 4 Pinwheels
2 8-ounce low fat cream cheese, softened
½ cup green onion, finely chopped
½ 4-ounce can green chili pepper, chopped
¼ cup jalapeño, finely chopped
1 package flour tortillas, 10-12 count

Directions:
1. Mix cream cheese, green onions and both peppers.
2. Spread on flour tortillas, roll and cut into slices.

Nutrition Facts (per serving)
Calories 64 Carbohydrates 7 g
Protein 2 g Dietary Fiber 0 g
Fat 0 g Sodium 162 mg Potassium 63 mg
Phosphorus 38 mg

CREAM CHEESE & ONION DIP

Ingredients:
Yield: 2 servings Serving size: ¼ cup
1 cucumber, seeds removed and grated
1 3-ounce package cream cheese, softened
2 tablespoons onion, grated
1 dash Tabasco® sauce
1 tablespoon mayonnaise

1 3-ounce package cream cheese, softened
2 tablespoons onion, grated
1 dash Tabasco® sauce
1 tablespoon mayonnaise

Directions:

1. Blend ingredients together.
2. Spread on bread or on unsalted crackers.
3. Garnish with paprika or green pepper slices.

Nutrition Facts (per serving)
Calories 219 Carbohydrates 6 g
Protein 4 g Dietary Fiber 1 g
Fat 21 g Sodium 185mg
Potassium 264 mg Phosphorus 80 mg

CRAB CAKES WITH LIME GINGER SAUCE

Ingredients:
Yield: 8 servings Serving size: 1
1/2 cup celery, finely diced
1/2 cup onion, finely diced
1 medium red bell pepper, finely diced
3 cups crab meat, well drained
2 eggs
1 cup mayonnaise
1/2 lemon lemon juice
1 teaspoon worcestershire sauce
1/2 teaspoon hot pepper sauce
1 tablespoon chives, minced
1 teaspoon fresh thyme, minced
1 teaspoon fresh garlic, minced
3/4 cup panko crumbs
1 recipe lime ginger sauce

Directions

1. In a large bowl, gently fold together all ingredients except the panko.
2. Generously sprinkle some panko on a baking sheet.
3. Scoop out mounds of crab mixture with an ice cream scoop and place on prepared baking sheet.
4. One by one, dredge mounds in panko, shaping into cakes as you go.
5. Cover and refrigerate.
6. Heat some oil in a nonstick skillet over medium-high heat.
7. Add crab cakes and saute' until golden brown and heated through, about 4 minutes per side.
8. Remove to paper towels and drain.
9. Prepare Lime Ginger Sauce per recipe and serve on the side

Nutrition Facts (per serving)
Calories 354 Carbohydrates 18 g
Protein 12 g Sodium 444 mg
Potassium 279 mg Phosphorus 133 mg

SWEET POTATO BURRITO

Ingredients:
Yield: 8 servings Serving size: 1
2 each sweet potato
2 each red bell peppers
1 teaspoon vegetable oil
1 small onion, diced
2 cloves garlic, crushed
1/2 teaspoon cumin
1 teaspoon chili powder
2 1/4 teaspoon onion powder
1 1/4 teaspoon garlic powder
1 can (15 ounces), low sodium black beans
1/2 cup vegetable stock to taste ground

pepper
8- 6 inch flour tortillas
3 green onions, sliced
1 cup shredded cheese or soy cheese
1/2 cup sour cream or soy sour cream
Directions:
1. Blend ingredients together.
2. Spread on bread or on unsalted crackers.
3. Garnish with paprika or green pepper slices.

Nutrition Facts (per serving)
Calories 219 Carbohydrates 6 g
Protein 4 g Dietary Fiber 1 g
Fat 21 g Sodium 185mg
Potassium 264 mg Phosphorus 80 mg

LOUISIANA BBQ SHRIMP

Ingredients:
Yield: 15 servings Serving size: 1
7.5 pounds shrimp
2 sticks butter
1 cup olive oil
1/2 cup chili sauce
1/4 cup Worcestershire sauce
2 lemon, thinly sliced
4 garlic cloves, minced
1/4 cup lemon juice
1 tablespoon parsley minced
2 teaspoons paprika
2 teaspoons oregano
2 teaspoons rosemary
3 teaspoons cayenne pepper
1 teaspoon Tabasco sauce
Directions:
1. Peel, devein, and wash shrimp.
2. Combine remaining ingredients in sauce pan.
3. Place over low heat and simmer for 30 minutes.
4. Lightly saute shrimp in olive oil until half cooked.
5. Pour BBQ sauce over shrimp and bring to a light boil.
6. Serve in a bread bowl or a regular bowl with plenty of french bread.

Nutrition Facts (per serving)
Calories 420 Carbohydrates 6 g
Protein 35 g Dietary Fiber 29 g
Sodium 666 mg Potassium 423 mg
Phosphorus 244 mg

STRAWBERRY SORBET

Ingredients:
Yield: 2 ½ cups Serving size: 6-ounces or ¾ cups
¼ cup sugar
1 cup frozen or fresh strawberries, cleaned
1 tablespoon lemon juice
¼ cup water
1 ¼ cups crushed or cubed ice
Directions:
1. Place ice in a blender.
2. Add all other ingredients, turn speed to crush or liquefy.

Nutrition Facts (per serving)
Calories 67 Carbohydrates 21 g
Protein 0 g Dietary Fiber 1 g Fat 16 g
Sodium 1 mg Potassium 79 mg
Phosphorus 12 mg

CRANBERRY PUNCH

Ingredients:
Yield: 46 servings Serving size: 6-ounces or ¾ cups
3 quarts cranberry juice
3 quarts pineapple juice
1 quart lemonade, frozen, undiluted
1 quart water 3
28-ounce bottles ginger ale
Directions:
1. Mix all ingredients together.
2. Chill and serve.

Nutrition Facts (per serving)
Calories 130 Carbohydrates 34 g
Protein 1 g Dietary Fiber 0 g Fat 0 g
Sodium 8 mg Potassium 153 mg
Phosphorus 16 mg

HOT SPICED APPLE JUICE

Ingredients:
Yield: 8 servings Serving size: ½ cup
½ teaspoon nutmeg
12 whole cloves
4 cinnamon sticks, broken
¼ teaspoon allspice
1 quart unsweetened apple
Directions:
1. Place all ingredients in saucepan.
2. Slowly bring to boil and let simmer for 20 minutes.
3. Strain and serve in cups.

Nutrition Facts (per serving)
Calories 63 Carbohydrates 15 g
Protein 1 g Dietary Fiber 1 g Fat 0 g

Sodium 6 mg Potassium 132 mg
Phosphorus 10 mg

BISCUITS WITH MASTER MIX

Ingredients:
Based on 12 servings per recipe.
3 cups (our recipe Master Mix)
2/3 cup Water
Directions:
1. Preheat oven to 450 degrees.
2. Combine ingredients and blend well.
3. Let stand 5 minutes.
4. On lightly floured board, knead dough about 15 times.
5. Roll out to 1/2 inch thickness and cut with flour cutter until you have 12 biscuits.
6. Place 2 inches apart on ungreased baking sheet.
7. Bake 10-12 minutes until golden brown.

Nutrition Facts (per serving)
Calories 174 Carbohydrates 18 g
Protein 3 g Dietary Fiber 10 g
Sodium 171 mg Potassium 81 mg
Phosphorus 51 mg

YEAST DINNER ROLLS

Ingredients:
Yield: 20 servings Serving size: 1 roll
1 cup hot water
6 tablespoons vegetable shortening
½ cup sugar

1 package yeast
2 tablespoons of warm water 1
egg 3 ¾-4 cups all-purpose flour

Directions:

1. Preheat oven to 400°F.
2. Combine hot water, shortening, and sugar in a large bowl. Set aside to cool to room temperature.
3. Dissolve yeast in warm water.
4. Add egg, yeast, and half the flour to the mixture in the large bowl. Beat well.
5. Stir in the remaining flour with a spoon until easy to handle.
6. Place dough in a greased bowl; grease top and cover top with plastic wrap.
7. Allow to rest 1 to 1 ½ hours or until the dough has doubled in size.
8. Cut off amount needed to shape rolls.
9. Bake rolls for 12 minutes or until done.

Nutrition Facts (per serving)
Calories 148 Carbohydrates 24 g
Protein 3 g Dietary Fiber 1 g
Sodium 5 mg Potassium 31 mg
Phosphorus 32 mg

GIBLET GRAVY

Ingredients:
Yield: 32 servings Serving size: 1 tablespoon
2 cups chicken broth (homemade from boiled chicken)
1 tablespoon all-purpose flour
1 hard boiled egg, sliced or chopped
1-2 poultry liver or giblets, boiled, chopped

Directions:

1. Stir 1 tablespoon of broth with flour until smooth.
2. Add remaining broth andcook over low heat, stirring constantly.
3. Add boiled egg and giblets.
4. Continue to stir until desired thickness (about 5 minutes).

Nutrition Facts (per serving)
Calories 13 Carbohydrates 1 g
Protein 1 g Dietary Fiber 0 g
Sodium 13 mg Potassium 31 mg
Phosphorus 16 mg

HERB RICE CASSEROLE

Ingredients:
Yield: 8 servings Serving size: ½ cup
1 cup white rice, uncooked
2 cups chicken stock, unsalted
¼ cup green bell pepper, chopped
½ teaspoon parsley flakes
1 tablespoon vegetable oil
3 Fresh green onions, chopped
1 tablespoon chives

Directions:

1. Preheat oven to 350°F.
2. Combine all ingredients, and place in casserole dish.
3. Bake in covered casserole for 45-50 minutes or until liquid is absorbed.

Nutrition Facts (per serving)
Calories 53 Carbohydrates 7 g
Protein 2 g Dietary Fiber 0 g Fat 2 g
Sodium 7 mg Potassium 74 mg
Phosphorus 29 mg

RICE O'BRIEN

Ingredients:
Yield: 4 servings Serving size: ½ cup
1½ cup water
1 cup rice, uncooked
½ cup onion, thinly sliced or chopped
¼ cup green pepper, chopped
¼ cup carrots, shredded
¼ teaspoon red pepper
½ teaspoon black pepper
½ teaspoon thyme or rosemary
1 tablespoon lemon juice
1 tablespoon margarine
Directions:
1. In a large saucepan with water boiling, combine all ingredients.
2. Let simmer in
covered pan for 15 minutes (do not stir).
3. Remove from pan; fluff rice lightly with fork.

Nutrition Facts (per serving)
Calories 207 Carbohydrates 40 g
Protein 4 g Dietary Fiber 1 g Fat 3 g
Sodium 32 mg Potassium 125 mg
Phosphorus 64 mg

OLD FASHIONED PANCAKES

Ingredients:
Yield: 4 small pancakes Serving size: 1 pancake
½ cup all purpose flour
1 egg, beaten
¼ cup granulated sugar
¼ teaspoon baking powder
¼ cup 2% milk plus

¼ cup water
1 tablespoon vegetable oil
Directions:
1. Combine first four ingredients in a bowl. Mix well. Add milk and water. Add more water for thinner pancakes or less for thicker pancakes.
2. Heat oil in a skillet or on a griddle. Pour ¼ cup batter on griddle. Cook until brown, turning on each side.

Nutrition Facts (per serving)
Calories 165 Carbohydrates 26 g
Protein 4 g Dietary Fiber 0 g Fat 5 g
Sodium 58 mg Potassium 57 mg
Phosphorus 64 mg

CORNBREAD DRESSING

Yield: 15 servings Serving size: 2" x 2" square or ¾ cup

Cornbread
Ingredients for cornbread
2 cups cornmeal (plain)
1 ½ cups all-purpose flour
2 ½ cups water
1 egg
2 tablespoons vegetable oil
Directions for cornbread
1. Preheat oven to 425ºF.
2. Combine cornmeal, flour, sugar, and baking powder in mixing bowl ; mix well.
3. Add water, egg and oil, mixing well.
4. Place in a 9" x 9" square greased baking pan.
5. Bake until golden brown.
6. When done, let cool, then crumble. Set aside to combine with

dressing ingredients.

Dressing

Ingredients for dressing

2 cups chicken parts and giblets
4 cups water
1 cup chopped onion
½ cup chopped celery
½ cup chopped green peppers
1 teaspoon black pepper
1 teaspoon poultry seasoning ù
1 teaspoon onion powder
1 teaspoon sage

Directions for dressing

1. Wash chicken parts and giblets and add to water in a large pot.
2. Add onion, celery, green pepper and black pepper.
3. Boil for 30 minutes until tender
4. When done, reserve 2 cups of broth for dressing (remaining broth may be used for giblet gravy on the following page). Let meat cool.
5. Remove meat from bone and add to remaining dressing ingredients.
6. Mix all ingredients together with 2 cups broth from chicken until mixture is moist.
7. Spread into baking pan.
8. Bake at 425ºF until golden brown.

Nutrition Facts (per serving)
Calories 156 Carbohydrates 29 g
Protein 4 g Dietary Fiber 2 g Fat 3 g
Sodium 75 mg Potassium 88 mg
Phosphorus 62 mg

HIGH PROTEIN BREAD

Ingredients:
Based on 16 servings per recipe.

3 cups whole wheat flour
1 cup all-purpose flour
1/2 cup wheat gluten
2 tablespoons sugar
1/2 teaspoon salt
2 tablespoons yeast
1/3 cup honey
1 1/2 teaspoons canola oil
2 cups warm water, 95-105 degrees

Directions:

1. Mix flours, gluten, and sugar in a mixing bowl.
2. In a seperate bowl, mix yeast, honey, and oil into the water.
3. Let stand and stir a bit until the yeast is dissolved, about 5 minutes.
4. Mix the yeast mixture into the flour mix to create the dough.
5. Knead the dough until you have elastic consistancy, adding more flour to the board as needed. Usually this take about 5 minutes.
6. Place the dough in a clean, lightly oiled bowl and cover with a towel. Leave it alone until it doubles in size. Dependent upon heat and humidity, this will take 45 minutes to an hour.
7. Pre-heat oven to 350 degrees and spray your 5×9 pan with oil.
8. Punch down dough and place in your pan.
9. Let it rise again just to the top of the pan. This could take anywhere from 30 minutes to an hour.
10. Place in oven for 50-55 minutes, the bread should have a rich brown color and should have a hollow sound when you tap it. Internal temperature should be around 200 degrees.

11. Remove loaf from the pan a after it is

slightly cooled. Let the loaf cool on a rack before slicing.

Nutrition Facts (per serving)
Calories 164 Carbohydrates 31 g
Protein 9 g Sodium 77 mg Potassium
101 mg Phosphorus 108 mg

BLUEBERRY BAKED BREAD

Ingredients:
Yield: 6 servings Serving size: ½ cup
1 quart blueberries, fresh or frozen
¼ cup water (omit if berries are frozen)
1 teaspoon lemon juice
½ cup sugar
1 pinch nutmeg
1 pinch cinnamon
1 tablespoon margarine
3 slices bread, buttered and
sprinkledwith cinnamon and sugar on
both sides
Directions:
1. Heat oven to 425ºF.
2. Wash blueberries
under cool running water.
3. Combine all ingredients in a saucepan
except bread. Bring to a boil.
4. Pour blueberry mixture into a shallow
baking pan; top with bread cut in halves.
5. Bake until brown (about 10 minutes).

Nutrition Facts (per serving)
Calories 176 Carbohydrates 39 g
Protein 2 g Dietary Fiber 3 g Fat 3 g
Sodium 92 mg Potassium 83 mg
Phosphorus 20 mg

WHITE BREAD DRESSING

Ingredients:
Yield: 4 servings Serving size: ½ cup
2 tablespoons margarine
¼ cup chopped onions
1 ½ cups plain bread crumbs or
3 slices bread, crumbled
¼ cup chopped celery
1 teaspoon poultry seasoning
¼ teaspoon garlic powder
¼ cup unsalted chicken broth
Directions:
1. Melt margarine in a small skillet. Add
onions. Stir until onions are tender.
2. Add bread crumbs, stirring constantly
to prevent scorching.
3. Remove from heat.
Add celery, poultry seasoning, garlic
powder and chicken broth.
4. Blend well. Place in a small baking pan.
5. Bake for 30 minutes at 375ºF.
6. If dressing appears too dry, add water
as needed.

Nutrition Facts (per serving)
Calories 107 Carbohydrates 11 g
Protein 2 g Dietary Fiber 1 g Fat 6 g
Sodium 129 mg Potassium 77 mg
Phosphorus 30 mg

BLUEBERRY MUFFINS

Ingredients:
Yield: 12 muffins Serving size: 1 muffin
1 egg white
¼ cup margarine
½ cup sugar

7 tablespoons water
½ teaspoon vanilla
extract
1 teaspoon baking powder
1 cup all-purpose flour
1 cup blueberries, canned and drained or
fresh
Directions:
1. Preheat oven to 375ºF.
2. Beat egg white in a small mixing bowl
until stiff. Set aside.
3. Cream margarine and sugar together
until smooth.
4. Add water and vanilla, mixing
thoroughly.
5. Add baking powder and flour.
6. Fold in beaten egg white and
blueberries.
7. Bake in greased muffin pan for 30
minutes.

Nutrition Facts (per serving)
Calories 123 Carbohydrates 21 g
Protein 1,5 g Dietary Fiber 1 g Fat 0 g
Sodium 139 mg Potassium 71 mg
Phosphorus 94 mg

BAKING POWDER BISCUITS

Ingredients:
Yield: 10 biscuits Serving size: 1 biscuit
2 cups all-purpose flour, sifted
3 teaspoons double acting baking
powder
2 teaspoons sugar
⅓ cup vegetable shortening
¼ cup 1% milk
½ cup water
Directions:

1. Pre-heat oven at 350ºF.
2. Sift dry ingredients into a bowl.
3. Cut in shortening until coarse crumbs
 form. Make a well in the mixture.
4. Pour milk and water into the well.
5. Stir quickly with a fork until dough
follows fork around the bowl.
6. Dough should be soft. Turn dough onto
fightly floured surface.
7. Knead gently 10-12 times. Roll or pat
dough until ½" thick.
8. Dip a 2 ½" biscuit cutter into flour; then
cut out 10 biscuits.
9. Bake biscuits on ungreased baking
sheet for 12-15 minutes.

Nutrition Facts (per serving)
Calories 162 Carbohydrates 21 g
Protein 3 g Dietary Fiber 1 g Fat 8 g
Sodium 150 mg Potassium 36 mg
Phosphorus 62 mg

FRENCH TOAST

Ingredients:
Yield: 4 servings Serving size: 1 slice
4 large egg whites, slightly beaten
¼ cup 1% milk
½ teaspoon cinnamon
¼ teaspoon allspice
4 slices white bread (may be toasted)
1 tablespoon margarine
Directions:
1. Add milk, cinnamon and allspice to
egg whites.
2. Dip bread into batter one
piece at a time.
3. Place on heated grill or

in skillet with melted margarine.
4. Turn bread after it is golden brown.
5. Serve hot with syrup (sugar free if diabetic).

Nutrition Facts (per serving)
Calories 125 Carbohydrates 14 g
Protein 7 g Dietary Fiber 1 g Fat 5 g
Sodium 194 mg Potassium 128 mg
Phosphorus 61 mg

HERB BREAD

Ingredients:
Yield: 1 loaf — about 15 slice Serving size:
1 slice
1 loaf french bread
¼ cup margarine (unsalted)
2 tablespoons chopped green onions
1 teaspoon thyme
¼ teaspoon tarragon
1 teaspoon basil flakes (optional)
½ teaspoon crushed marjoram (optional)
Directions:
1. Heat oven to 350ºF.
2. Slice french bread almost to the bottom crust.
3. Combine margarine with remaining ingredients.
4. Spread butter mixture on cut surfaces or slices. May use a brush.
5. Place on a baking sheet or pan.
6. Bake for 15-20 minutes.

Nutrition Facts (per serving)
Calories 120 Carbohydrates 18 g
Protein 4 g Dietary Fiber 1 g Fat 4 g
Sodium 208 mg Potassium 44 mg
Phosphorus 30 mg

HOMEMADE PAN SAUSAGE

Ingredients:
Yield: 12 servings Serving size: 1 patty
1 pound fresh lean ground pork, beef, chicken or turkey.
2 teaspoons ground sage
2 teaspoons granulated sugar
1 teaspoon ground black pepper
½ teaspoon ground red pepper
1 teaspoon basil (optional) cooking spray
Directions:
1. Ask the butcher to grind the pork roast or beef loin of your choice.
2. To make sausage, mix all ingredients well.
3. Measure 2 tablespoons of meat mixture and make into a patty.
4. Pan fry or broil until thoroughly cooked.

Nutrition Facts (per serving)
Calories 96 Carbohydrates 1 g
Protein 6 g Dietary Fiber 0 g Fat 7 g
Sodium 22 mg Potassium 87 mg
Phosphorus 53 mg

MAPLE SAUSAGE

Ingredients:
Based on 12 servings per recipe.
1 pound ground pork or beef
1/2 pound ground turkey
1/2 teaspoon black pepper
3/4 teaspoon dried sage (or 2 tablespoons fresh)
1/4 teaspoon mace or nutmeg
1/4 teaspoon ground all spice
2 teaspoons maple syrup

1 teaspoon water

Directions:

1. Mix all ingredients in a large bowl.
2. Refrigerate for at least 4 hours, or overnight.
3. Form into patties and cook in skillet over medium-high heat until well browned, or about 10 minutes.

Nutrition Facts (per serving)

Calories 96 Carbohydrates 1 g
Protein 6 g Dietary Fiber 0 g Fat 7 g
Sodium 22 mg Potassium 87 mg
Phosphorus 53 mg

PUMPKIN SPICED APPLESAUCE BREAD OR MUFFINS

Ingredients:

Yield: 12 servings Serving size: 1 patty
1 pound fresh lean ground pork, beef, chicken or turkey.
2 teaspoons ground sage
2 teaspoons granulated sugar
1 teaspoon ground black pepper
½ teaspoon ground red pepper
1 teaspoon basil (optional) cooking spray

Directions:

1. Preheat oven to 350 degrees.
2. Grease loaf or muffin pan.
3. In a medium bowl, whisk applesauce, brown sugar, oil, and eggs together.
4. In a seperate medium bowl, mix remaining ingredients.
5. Add applesauce mixture to flour mixture and stir until just combined (careful not to over mix).
6. Place batter in loaf or muffin pan.

7. If baking a loaf, bake for about 50-60 minutes.
8. If baking muffins, bake for about 20 minutes.
9. You can test doneness by poking with a toothpick, which should come out clean.

Nutrition Facts (per serving)

Calories 252 Carbohydrates 38 g
Protein 3 g Dietary Fiber 10 g
Sodium 141 mg Potassium 82 mg
Phosphorus 41 mg

VEGETABLE OMELET

Ingredients:

Based on 1 serving per recipe.
2 eggs
2 tablespoons water
1 tablespoon unsalted butter
1/2 cup filling (vegetables, meat, seafood)

Directions:

1. Beat together eggs and water until blended.

2. In a 10-inch omelet pan or fry pan, heat butter until just hot enough to sizzle a drop of water.

3. Pour in egg mixture. Mixture should set at edges right away. With an inverted pancake turner, carefully push cooked portions at edges toward center so uncooked portions can reach the hot pan surface. Tilt pan and move as necessary.

4. Continue until egg is set and will not flow. Fill the omelet with 1/2 cup of vegetables, meat, or seafood filling, if

desired. Put filling on left side if you're right handed and the right side if you're left handed.

5. With the pancake turner, fold omelet in half. Invert onto a plate with the omelet's bottom side facing up.

Nutrition Facts (per serving)
Calories 255 Carbohydrates 1,3 g
Protein 13 g Dietary Fiber 2 g
Sodium 145 mg Potassium 122 mg
Phosphorus 195 mg

MEXICAN BRUNCH EGGS

Ingredients:
Based on 8 servings per recipe.
1/2 cup chopped onion
2 cloves garlic, crushed
2 tablespoons margarine
1 1/2 cups frozen corn, thawed
1 1/2 teaspoons ground cumin
1/8 teaspoon cayenne pepper
8 eggs, beaten
8 slices toasted bread
Directions:
1. In a large skillet, saute onion and garlic in margarine until onion is soft.
2. Add corn, cumin, and cayenne; stir to combine.
3. Pour in eggs or egg substitute and cook over low heat, stirring occasionally until eggs are set.
4. Arrange toast triangles on a large platter.
5. Spoon egg mixture on toast triangles.
6. Serve immediately.

Nutrition Facts (per serving)
Calories 214 Carbohydrates 13 g
Protein 9 g Dietary Fiber 14 g
Sodium 147 mg Potassium 240 mg
Phosphorus 91 mg

LOADED VEGGIE EGGS

Ingredients:
Yield: 2 servings Serving Size: 1/2 recipe
4 whole eggs
1 c cauliflower
3 c fresh spinach
1 garlic clove, minced
1/4 c bell pepper, chopped
1/4 cup onion, chopped
1/4 tsp black pepper
1 tbsp oil of choice (coconut or avocado oil is good for high heat)
fresh parsley and spring onion for garnish
*optional tomatoes on side if no potassium restriction
Directions:
1. Beat eggs with pepper until light and fluffy, set aside.
2. Heat oil over medium heat in large skillet.
3. Add onions and peppers to skillet and saute until peppers are translucent and golden.
4. Add garlic, stirring quickly to combine and immediately adding cauliflower and spinach.
5. Saute vegetables, turn heat to medium-low and cover for 5 minutes.
6. Add eggs, stirring to combine with vegetables.
7. When the eggs are cooked thoroughly, top with fresh parsley or spring onions.

If no potassium restriction can serve with a side of bright fresh tomatoes topped with cracker black pepper. A touch of feta or a strong sharp cheese would also be delicious with these
Note:
To reduce phosphorus further you can you 8 egg whites instead of egg yolks.

Nutrition Facts (per serving)
Calories 240 Carbohydrates 7,8 g
Protein 15 g Dietary Fiber 2,7 g Fat 4 g
Sodium 195 mg Potassium 605 mg
Phosphorus 254 mg

PANCAKES WITH MASTER MIX

Ingredients:
Based on 5 servings per recipe.
2 1/4 cups Master Mix (our Reipe)
1 tablespoon sugar
1 egg, beaten
1 1/2 cups milk
Directions:
1. Combine our Mater mix recipe and sugar in a medium bowl.
2. Combine egg and milk in a small bowl and add all at once to dry ingredients.
3. Blend well.
4. Let stand for 5-10 minutes.
5. Cook on a hot oiled grill about 3-4 minutes or until browned on both sides.

Nutrition Facts (per serving)
Calories 348 Carbohydrates 36 g
Protein 9 g Dietary Fiber 19 g
Sodium 302 mg Potassium 260 mg
Phosphorus 175 mg

JELLIED CRANBERRY SAUCE

Ingredients:
Yield: 16 servings Serving Size: 2 tablespoons
1 cup granulated sugar
12 ounces fresh whole cranberries
Directions:
1. In a medium saucepan combine sugar and 1 cup water; bring to a boil.
2. Add cranberries to water and return to a boil. Reduce the heat to medium and boil for 10 minutes while stirring occassionaly.
3. Pour cooked cranberries into a wire mesh strainer over a mixing bowl. Using the back of a spoon mash berries to force pulp into the bowl. Discard skins.
4. Stir sauce and pour into a serving bowl. Cool at room temperature, then chill in the refrigerator until ready to serve.

Nutrition Facts (per serving)
Calories 58 Carbohydrates 15 g
Protein 0 g Dietary Fiber 0,7 g Fat 0 g
Sodium 1 mg Potassium 16 mg
Phosphorus 2 mg

GINGERBREAD COOKIES

Ingredients:
1/4 Butter (Softened)
1/4c. 50% to 70% vegetable oil spread
1/2c. Packed brown sugar*
2tsp. Ground ginger
1tsp. Baking soda
1tsp. Ground cinnamon

1/4 tsp. Ground Cloves
1/4c. Full-flavor Molasses
1 Egg
2 1/2c. Almond Flour

Directions:

1. In a large bowl, combine butter and vegetable oil spread; beat with an electric mixer on medium to high speed for 30 seconds.
2. Add brown sugar, ginger, baking soda, cinnamon, salt, and cloves. Beat until well mixed, scraping side of bowl occasionally. Beat in molasses and egg. (Mixture will look curdled.)
3. Add flour, beating just until combined. Divide dough in half. Cover and chill the dough for 2 to 3 hours or until easy to handle.
4. Preheat oven to 375 degrees F. Lightly grease cookie sheets or line with parchment paper; set aside. On a lightly floured surface, roll dough, half at a time, to 1/8-inch thickness. Using a 2- to 3-inch gingerbread person cookie cutter, cut out shapes; reroll scraps as necessary. Place cutouts 1 inch apart on prepared cookie sheets.
5. Bake for 4 to 6 minutes or until edges are firm and centers are set. Cool on cookie sheets on wire racks for 1 minute. ransfer to wire racks; cool.Makes 36 (3-inch) cookies.

Nutrition Facts (per serving)
Calories 73 Carbohydrates 12 g
Protein 1 g Fat 2 g Sodium 4 mg
Potassium 130 mg Phosphorus 105 mg

ROASTED TURKEY

Ingredients:

Yield: 8 plus leftovers Serving Size: 3 ounces
12 pound turkey, fresh or frozen (avoid self-basting)
1 teaspoon poultry seasoning
4 sprigs fresh parsley
4 sprigs fresh sage
4 sprigs fresh rosemary
4 sprigs fresh thyme
1/2 cup unsalted butter
1 cup low-sodium turkey stock from turkey giblets

Directions:

1. Check plastic wrap on turkey to determine cooking time.
2. Preheat oven to 425° F. Remove neck and giblet bag from cavity of turkey. Rinse turkey with cold water, then pat dry with clean paper towels.
3. Using several fingers, loosen skin from turkey breast and drumsticks. Rub poultry seasoning onto turkey flesh under skin. Place parsley, sage, rosemary, and thyme sprigs between turkey skin and flesh.
4. Place a meat thermometer in the fleshy part of the thigh, without touching the bone.
5. Coat turkey with melted butter (or oil) and place breast side up in a roasting pan on a rack. Cover loosely with aluminum foil. Cook 30 minutes then reduce heat to 325° F.
6. Begin basting the turkey every 15 to 20 minutes with the giblet stock and pan juices. During last 30 minutes remove foil

from roasting pan. Cook for 3 to 4 hours until meat thermometer registers 165º F.
7. Let turkey rest 30 minutes before carving.

Nutrition Facts (per serving)
Calories 144 Carbohydrates 0 g
Protein 25 g Fat 4 g Sodium 57 mg
Potassium 256 mg Phosphorus 182 mg

COCONUT MARSHMALLOW SALAD

Ingredients:
Yield: 8 Serving Size: 3/4 cup
1 package (8.8 ounces) fruit flavored marshmallows
1 cup dried coconut, shredded
1 can (15 ounces) drained fruit cocktail
2 cups sour cream
Directions:
1. Mix all ingredients in a bowl.

2. Transfer to a glass bowl to serve.

3. If you like a creamy salad, refrigerate an hour before serving. If you like a molded salad, refrigerate overnight.

Nutrition Facts (per serving)
Calories 317 Carbohydrates 40 g
Protein 3 g Fiber 3 g Fat 18 g
Sodium 48 mg Potassium 185 mg
Phosphorus 74 mg

SPICED EGGNOG

Ingredients:
Yield: 6 plus leftovers Serving Size: 1/2 cup
2 cups half & half creamer
3/4 cup low cholesterol egg product
1/4 cup sugar
2 teaspoons rum extract
1/2 teaspoon pumpkin pie spice
1/4 teaspoon nutmeg
6 tablespoons whipped cream
Directions:
1. Combine the half & half creamer, egg product, sugar, rum extract and pumpkin pie spice in a chilled blender and blend for 1 to 2 minutes.

2. Pour into 6 small glasses. Top each serving with a tablespoon of whipped topping and a sprinkle of nutmeg.
Helpful hints:
Rum extract may be replaced with 2 tablespoons rum, if desired. Always check with your doctor before including alcohol in your diet.
Replace sugar with low-calorie sweetener to decrease carbohydrate to 4 grams and calories to 125 per serving.
Check half & half ingredients and avoid brands with phosphate additives.

Nutrition Facts (per serving)
Calories 162 Carbohydrates 13 g
Protein 5 g Fiber 0 g Fat 10 g
Sodium 78 mg Potassium 149 mg
Phosphorus 83 mg

GARLIC MASHED POTATOES

Ingredients:
Yield: 4 plus Serving Size: 1/2 cup
2 medium potatoes
2 garlic cloves
1/4 cup butter
1/4 cup 1% low fat milk

Directions:
1. Peel and slice the potatoes into small pieces.Double-boil to reduce potassium if you are on a low potassium diet. (see helpful hints.)
2. Boil potatoes and garlic over medium heat until soft.
3. Drain off cooking water.
4. Whip potatoes and garlic with beater, slowly adding butter and milk until whipped smooth.

Helpful hints:
Double the garlic for a stronger garlic flavor.
Potatoes are very high in potassium but you can remove part of the potassium by using one of these methods:
Double boil method: Peel and small dice potatoes. Place in a large pot of water and bring to a boil. Drain the water and add fresh water to the pot. Bring to a boil, cook for 10 minutes then drain and prepare as desired.
Leaching method: Peel and dice potatoes. Place in a large pot of warm tap water and soak for 2 to 4 hours. Drain and cook as desired.
Leached potatoes can be blanched and frozen in batches. To blanch vegetables, add to boiling water for one minute, remove and rinse in cold water before freezing.
*Potassium content taken from reference values for double-boiling small peeled and diced potatoes.

Nutrition Facts (per serving)
Calories 185 Carbohydrates 15 g
Protein 2 g Fat 13 g Fiber 0,7
Sodium 103 mg Potassium 205* mg
Phosphorus 65 mg

PUMPKIN PIE

Ingredients:
Yield: One 9" pie Serving Size: 1/8 slice
FILLING
2 3/4 cups pureed spaghetti squash
1/4 cup maple syrup
1/4 cup brown sugar
1/3 cup unsweetened plain almond milk
1 Tbsp olive oil, or melted coconut oil
2 1/2 Tbsp cornstarch or arrowroot powder
1 3/4 tsp pumpkin pie spice (or sub mix of ginger, cinnamon, nutmeg & cloves)
1/4 tsp sea salt
Your favorite crust (Our favorite crust is the low sodium pie crust)

Directions:
1. Preheat oven to 350 degrees F (176 C) and prepare pie filling.
2. Add all pie ingredients to a blender and blend until smooth, scraping down sides as needed. Taste and adjust seasonings as needed. Pour filling into pie crust and bake for 58-65 minutes. The crust should be light golden brown and the filling will still be just a bit jiggly and

have some cracks on the top. Remove from oven and let cool completely before loosely covering and transferring to the refrigerator to fully set for 4-6 hours, preferably overnight.

3. Slice and serve with your whipped topping of choice

Nutrition Facts (per serving)
Calories 195 Carbohydrates 26 g
Protein 2 g Fat 9,5 g Sodium 133 mg
Potassium 89 mg Phosphorus 21 mg

LIGHTER CHRISTMAS PUDDING

Ingredients:
Yield: 8 approx
1 1/2 cups raisins
1/2 cup dried papaya chunks
1/2 cup dried figs
1/2 cup dried apricots
1/2 cup dried cranberries
1/3 cup brandy
1 apple grated (approx 3/4 cup grated)
1 carrot large, or 2 small, grated (approx 3/4 -1 cup grated)
1 orange juice and zest ie from 1 orange
4 oz beef suet, or finely chopped or grated
4 oz fresh breadcrumbs
3/4 cup soft brown sugar, or 1/2 cup brown, 1/4 cup granulated
1/2 cup all purpose flour plain flour
3 eggs
1 tsp baking powder
1 tsp cinnamon
1/2 tsp nutmeg
1/4 tsp allspice

At least 1 day before needed
Chop the papaya chunks, figs (removing any tough stem) and apricots to roughly the same size as the raisins and mix all the dried fruit and brandy together. Leave overnight, stirring now and again so as much of the fruit as possible can soak up the brandy.

On day (or further ahead of time)
In a large bowl, mix the remaining ingredients - apple, carrot, orange juice and zest, suet, breadcrumbs, sugar, flour, eggs, baking powder and spices. The eggs can either be beaten separately first or put in last and break them up a bit before you combine everything.
Add the soaked dried fruit and mix well then transfer to a pudding bowl, pack down and smooth the top.
Cover the bowl with greaseproof/parchment paper, making a fold in the paper over the middle and tie string/twine around the paper to hold the paper on. Make a string handle and trim the paper - see picture above.
Place the bowl in a steamer - can improvise using a regular large pan and something to raise the bowl off the bottom - and steam for at least 3 1/2 hours, checking the water level occasionally to ensure it doesn't go dry. Once finished, allow to cool, remove the greaseproof/parchment paper and put on a new paper lid and store in a cool dark place until ready to use. It will keep for a good few weeks.

Before serving
When ready to use, steam again for at

least 2 to 2 1/2 hours, making a min of 7 hours in total.

Once it has finished steaming, remove the lid, loosen from the bowl and place a plate over the bowl. Tip over the plate and bowl so the pudding falls onto the plate, helping it as needed as you remove the bowl.

To serve, heat some brandy in a small pan, set light to the brandy and pour over the pudding.

Nutrition Facts (per serving)
Calories 550 Carbohydrates 82 g
Protein 6 g Fat 16 g Sodium 150 mg
Potassium 626 mg

EASY SHEPHERD'S PIE

Ingredients:
Yield: 8 portions Serving Size: 1/8 pie
1 medium onion
3/4 cup carrots
3 garlic cloves
2 medium potatoes
4 tablespoons butter
1-1/2 pounds lean ground beef (7% fat)
1/2 teaspoon black pepper
2 teaspoon Worcestershire sauce
1/3 cup tomato sauce
3/4 cup frozen green peas
1 cup 1% low-fat milk
1/2 cup brown gravy
Directions:
1. Chop onion and carrots. Mince garlic cloves. Peel potatoes and cut into 1/2 inch pieces. Boil in a large pot of water for 5 minutes. Drain water, replace with fresh water and boil again until potatoes are tender; drain.
2. While potatoes are cooking, melt 2 tablespoons butter in a large frying pan. Over medium heat, sauté onions and garlic until tender (10 minutes).
3. Add ground beef and sauté until no longer pink.
4. Add pepper, Worcestershire sauce, tomato sauce and vegetables. Simmer on low heat, uncovered, for 10 minutes.
5. Preheat oven to 400° F.
6. Mash potatoes in a bowl with 2 tablespoons of butter. Mix in milk to give potatoes a creamy consistency. Add pepper to taste.
7. Spread beef evenly in a baking dish. Cover evenly with mash potatoes. Use a fork to make a design.
8. Bake for 30 minutes until bubbly. To brown top, broil for 2 minutes if desired.
9. Serve 1 tablespoons of gravy over each portion.

Nutrition Facts (per serving)
Calories 390 Carbohydrates 22 g
Protein 26 g Fat 22 g Fiber 2,3 g
Sodium 312 mg Potassium 605 mg
Phosphorus 296 mg

FRIED APPLES

Ingredients:
Based on 5 serving per recipe
5 cups apples, peeled and sliced
2 teaspoons cinnamon
1 teaspoon vanilla
Directions:

1. Spray skillet with non stick coating.
2. Add apples.
3. Saute apple until soft.
4. Add cinnamon and vanill

Nutrition Facts (per serving)
Calories 94 Carbohydrates 1 g
Protein 0 g Sodium 1 mg
Potassium 153 mg Phosphorus 10 mg

RASPBERRY PEAR SORBET

Ingredients:
Yield: 6 Serving Serving Size: 1/2 cup
1/2 cup sugar
1 pint fresh raspberries
2 large pear halves, canned in juice
1/3 cup lime juice
1 tablespoon pear liqueur or vodka
(optional)
Fresh raspberries (optional)
Directions:
For simple syrup, in a small saucepan
bring 1 cup water and the sugar to
boiling, stirring to dissolve sugar. Reduce
heat. Simmer, uncovered, for 3 minutes.
Remove from heat. Place in refrigerator
to cool.
1. Meanwhile, for puree, in food processor
combine the 1 pint raspberries, pear,
lime juice, and pear liqueur. Cover;
process 30 seconds or until smooth. Stir
in chilled simple syrup.
2. Prepare per ice-cream maker
instructions OR spread mixture in an
8x8x2-inch baking pan. Cover; freeze 4
hours or until solid. Break up mixture
with a fork; place in food processor.
Cover; process 30 seconds or until

smooth. Transfer to 1-quart freezer
container; cover and freeze sorbet 6
to 8 hours or until solid. To serve, let
stand at room temperature 5 minutes
before scooping. Serve with additional
raspberries. Makes 6 (1/2-cup) servin.

Nutrition Facts (per serving)
Calories 135 Carbohydrates 32 g
Protein 1 g Fat 0,4 g Fiber 5
Sodium 3 mg Potassium 169 mg
Phosphorus 28 mg

BLUEBERRY SQUARES

Ingredients:
Based on 16 servings per recipe.
1 1/2 cups flour
1 cup oats
1 teaspoon cinnamon
1 cup sugar
3/4 cup or 1 1/2 sticks melted butter
(unsalted if you can)
3 cups blueberries
zest of 1 lemon
3 tablespoons cornstarch
3/4 cup sugar
1 cup water
Directions:
1. Preheat oven to 350 degrees.
2. In a medium bowl, combine flour,
oats, cinnamon, sugar, and butter until
crumbly.
3. Press 1/2 of the flour and oat mixture
into a 9 inch square pan.
4. Toss the blueberries with the lemon
zest and cover the bottom of the pan.
5. Mix together cornstarch and sugar in
a microwave safe bowl, gradually stir in

water and heat until just boiling.

6. Pour water/cornstarch/sugar mixture over the blueberries.

7. Pour the rest of the flour/oat mixture over the top.

8. Cook for 45 minutes-1 hour.

Nutrition Facts (per serving)
Calories 247 Carbohydrates 40 g
Protein 2 g Sodium 3 mg
Potassium 38 mg Phosphorus 17 mg

SCARLET'S FROZEN FANTASY

Ingredients:
Yield: 4 servings Serving size: 4-ounces
1 cup cranberry juice cocktail
1 cup fresh whole strawberries, washed and hulled
2 tablespoons fresh lime juice
¼ cup sugar
8-9 ice cubes strawberries for garnishing

Directions:
1. Combine cranberry juice, strawberries, lime juice and sugar in a blender. Mix well.

2. Add ice cubes and blend until smooth.

3. Pour into chilled glasses and garnish with a fresh strawberry.

Nutrition Facts (per serving)
Calories 100 Carbohydrates 24 g
Protein 0 g Sodium 3 mg Fat 0 Fiber 1 g
Potassium 109 mg Phosphorus 129 mg

RHUBARB SQUARES

Ingredients:
Based on 12 servings per recipe.
1 cup all-purpose flour
3/4 cup oatmeal
1 teaspoon cinnamon
1 cup brown sugar
1/2 cup unsalted butter, melted
4 cups rhubarb, chopped
1 cup granulated sugar
1 cup water
3 tablespoons cornstarc

Directions:
1. Preheat oven to 350 degrees.

2. Mix flour, oatmeal, cinnamon and brown sugar together.

3. Add melted butter and mix until crumbly.

4. Press 2/3 of the mixture into 9×9 inch square pan.

5. Cover with rhubarb.

6. Combine sugar, water and cornstarch in a small saucepan; bring to a boil for one minute or until thickened.

7. Pour over rhubarb.

8. Sprinkle remaining crumb mixture on top.

9. Bake for 1 hour.

10. Cut into 12 squares.

Nutrition Facts (per serving)
Calories 251 Carbohydrates 44 g
Protein 2 g Sodium 8 mg
Potassium 192 mg Phosphorus 46 mg

JEWELED COOKIES

Ingredients:
Yield: 50 cookies Serving size: 2 cookies.
½ cup softened unsalted butter or margarine
1 cup brown sugar, packed
1 medium egg
¼ cup milk
1 teaspoon vanilla
1 ¾ cups all-purpose flour, sifted
1 teaspoon baking powder
15 large gumdrops, chopped

Directions:
1. Preheat oven to 400°F.
2. Cream butter, sugar and egg thoroughly.
3. Stir in milk and vanilla.
4. Mix flour with baking powder in a separate bowl. Add to above ingredients.
5. Mix in gumdrops and chill dough for at least one hour.
6. Drop dough by tablespoonfuls onto greased cookie sheet.
7. Bake 8-10 minutes until golden brown.

Nutrition Facts (per serving)
Calories 104 Carbohydrates 22 g
Protein 1 g Sodium 9 mg Fat 0 Fiber 0
Potassium 29 mg Phosphorus 16 mg

FRUIT SALAD

Ingredients:
Yield: 10 servings Serving size: ½ cup
2 cups canned fruit cocktail, drained
1 cup canned pineapple chunks, drained
1 cup whole or sliced strawberries, hulled
1 cup apple, peeled, cored and diced
1 cup marshmallows ½ cup non-dairy whipped topping margarine
1 cup brown sugar, packed
1 medium egg
¼ cup milk
1 teaspoon vanilla
1 ¾ cups all-purpose flour, sifted
1 teaspoon baking powder
15 large gumdrops, chopped

Directions:
1. Combine all fruits together.
2. Add marshmallows and whipped topping; mix well.
3. Refrigerate and serve chilled.

Nutrition Facts (per serving)
Calories 57 Carbohydrates 14 g
Protein 1 g Sodium 9 mg Fat 0 Fiber 1 g
Potassium 120 mg Phosphorus 15 mg

LEMON CRISPIES

Ingredients:
Yield: 5 dozen Serving size: 2 cookies
1 cup unsalted butter or margarine
1 cup granulated sugar
1 egg
1 ½ teaspoons lemon extract
1 ½ cup all-purpose flour, sifted

Directions:
1. Preheat oven to 375°F.
2. Cream butter with sugar.
3. Add egg and lemon extract, beat until light and fluffy.
4. Add flour, mix until smooth.

5. Drop batter by level tablespoon onto ungreased cookie sheet,at least 2" apart.
6. Bake for 10 minutes until brown around the edges.
7. Remove from cookie sheet after the cookies have cooled for a minute.

Nutrition Facts (per serving)
Calories 115 Carbohydrates 12 g
Protein 2 g Sodium 12 mg Fat 6 Fiber 0 g
Potassium 20 mg Phosphorus 23 mg

FRUIT IN THE CLOUDS

Ingredients:
Yield: 4 squares Serving size: 1 square (2" x 2")
1 can fruit cocktail, drained
1 can mandarin orange, drained
8 ounces whipped cream, frozen
Directions:
1. Mix all ingredients together.
2. Freeze in8" x 8" container or individual molds.

Nutrition Facts (per serving)
Calories 113 Carbohydrates 23 g
Protein 1 g Sodium 20 mg Fat 3 Fiber 0 g
Potassium 152 mg Phosphorus 29 mg

CREAM CHEESE COOKIES

Ingredients:
Yield: 7 dozen cookies Serving size: 1 cookie
1 cup butter or margarine, softened
1 3-ounce package cream cheese, softened
1 cup sugar
1 egg yolk
2 ½ cups all-purpose flour
1 teaspoon vanilla extract candied cherry halves
Directions:
1. Preheat oven to 325°F.
2. Cream butter
and cream cheese; slowly add sugar, beating until fluffy.
3. Beat in egg yolk;
add flour and vanilla, mix well.
4. Chill dough at least one hour
5. Shape dough into 1" balls; place on greased cookie sheets.
6. Gently press a cherry half into each cookie.
7. Bake for 12-15 minutes.

Nutrition Facts (per serving)
Calories 80 Carbohydrates 11 g
Protein 0,5 g Sodium 31 mg Fat 4 g
Fiber 0 g Potassium 15 mg
Phosphorus 14 mg

BAKED EGG CUSTARD

Ingredients:
Yield: 4 servings Serving size: ½ cup
2 medium eggs
¼ cup 2% milk
3 tablespoons sugar
1 teaspoon vanilla or lemon extract
1 teaspoon nutmeg
Directions:
1. Preheat oven to 325°F.
2. Combine all ingredients, and beat for

one minute withelectric mixture until thoroughly mixed.

3. Pour into custard cups or muffin pans.

4. Sprinkle nutmeg on top.

5. Bake 20-30 minutes or until knife inserted into the center of the custard comes out clean.

Nutrition Facts (per serving)
Calories 70 Carbohydrates 9 g
Protein 3 g Sodium 34 mg Fat 3 g
Fiber 0 g Potassium 30 mg
Phosphorus 42 mg

SPICED POUND CAKE

Ingredients:
Yield: 16 slices Serving size: 1 slice
3 sticks butter or margarine
1 ¼ teaspoons ground nutmeg or mace
1 teaspoon vanilla extract
1 pound sifted powdered sugar
6 eggs
3 cups cake flour powdered sugar
Directions:
1. Preheat oven to 325°F.
2. Cream butter in a large bowl until softened.
3. Blend in nutmeg or mace and vanilla extract.
4. Gradually stir in powdered sugar.
5. Add eggs, one at a time, beating well after each addition.
6. Gradually stir in flour.
7. Grease only the bottom and lightly flour a 10" x 4" round tube pan. Note: do not grease the sides!
8. Bake for 1 hour and 20 minutes or until a cake tester inserted in the center comes out clean.

9. Allow cake to cool. Sprinkle with powdered sugar when cold.

Nutrition Facts (per serving)
Calories 174 Carbohydrates 33 g
Protein 3 g Sodium 45 mg Fat 5 g
Fiber 0 g Potassium 51 mg
Phosphorus 25 mg

SPRITZ COOKIES

Ingredients:
Yield: 75 cookies Serving size: 2 cookies
5 cups all-purpose flour
2 cups butter
1 cup plus
2 tablespoons sugar
2 eggs
1 teaspoon almond extract
2 teaspoons vanilla extract
Directions:
1. Preheat oven to 400°F.
2. Combine flour, butter and sugar.
3. Add eggs and extracts; mix with a spoon or hand mixer on low speed.
4. Drop cookies onto ungreased baking sheet or use cookie gun.
5. Bake for 5-8 minutes.
6. Cool and serve

Nutrition Facts (per serving)
Calories 172 Carbohydrates 26 g
Protein 2 g Sodium 56 mg Fat 4 g
Fiber 0 g Potassium 29 mg
Phosphorus 22 mg

FRUIT CRUNCH (CRUMB PIE)

Ingredients:
Yield: 8 servings Serving size: ½ cup
4 large tart apples, pared, cored and sliced
¾ cup sugar
½ cups all-purpose flour, sifted
⅓ cup margarine, softened
¾ cup rolled oats
¾ teaspoon nutmeg

Directions:
1. Preheat oven to 375°F.
2. Place apples in a greased 8" square pan.
3. Combine remaining ingredients in a medium bowl,and spread over fruit.
4. Bake 30-35 minutes or until fruit is tender and lightly browned.

Nutrition Facts (per serving)
Calories 217 Carbohydrates 36 g
Protein 1,4 g Sodium 62 mg Fat 2 g
Fiber 2 g Potassium 68 mg
Phosphorus 37 mg

RIBBON CAKES

Ingredients:
Yield: 84 cookies Serving size: 2 cookies
3 cups unsifted all-purpose flour
1 cup sugar
1 teaspoon baking powder
1 cup (½ pound) butter or margarine, softened
2 whole eggs plus
1 egg white
½ teaspoon vanilla
1 cup jelly or jam (plum blackberry, or raspberry jelly, or apricot jam)
2 tablespoons sugar

Directions:
1. Heat oven to 375°F.
2. In a large bowl, combine flour, sugar, and baking powder.
3. Blend in butter with finger tips or pastry blender until mixture resembles cornmeal.
4. Add eggs, egg white and vanilla; work into stiff dough.
5. Divide dough into two balls, one twice the size ofthe other. On a heavily floured board (¼to ½ cup flour), roll out the larger ball to 1/8" thickness.
6. Place rolled dough in a cookie pan (11" x 15 ½"), smoothing out to edges and patching corners. Spread jelly over the top.
7. Roll out remaining dough to 1/8" thickness and cut into ½ " wide strips; place strips diagonally acrossthe jelly, ½" apart. Sprinkle sugar over the top. Place in oven.
8. When edges start to brown (about 20 minutes), take pan from the oven, cut off and remove about a 3" strip all around the edges. Return pan to oven, remove after 10 minutes.
9. Cut into 1" x 2" rectangles. Makes 7 dozen cookies.

Nutrition Facts (per serving)
Calories 106 Carbohydrates 15 g
Protein 1 g Sodium 65 mg Fat 5 g
Fiber 0 g Potassium 17 mg
Phosphorus 27 mg

CHOCOLATE - ORANGE RAISIN COOKIES

Ingredients:
Based on 36 servings per recipe.
3 cups all-purpose flour
1 cup unsweetened cocoa powder
1 tablespoon baking powder, low sodium
1 1/3 cups margarine
1/4 cup powdered artificial sweetener
4 eggs
2/3 cup orange juice
2 cups raisins

Directions:
1. Preheat oven to 375 degrees.
2. Sift together flour, cocoa and baking powder.
3. Using a stand or hand mixer, beat margarine until creamy; beat in artificial sweetner.
4. Add eggs and beat well.
5. Add dry ingredients alternately with orange juice.
6. Stir in raisins.
7. Drop cookie dough by teaspoonfuls on ungreased baking sheets.
8. Bake for 10 minutes.
9. Remove and let cool

Nutrition Facts (per serving)
Calories 141 Carbohydrates 17 g
Protein 2 g Sodium 66 mg Fiber 8 g
Potassium 139 mg Phosphorus 52 mg

STRAWBERRIES BRULEE

Ingredients:
Based on 8 servings per recipe.
2, 3 ounce packages cream cheese, softened
1 cup sour cream
1/4 cup + 2 tablespoons brown sugar, packed and divided
1 quart fresh strawberries

Directions:
1. In bowl, beat cream cheese with electric mixer until fluffy.
2. Add sour cream and two tablespoons brown sugar; beat till smooth.
3. Reserve 1 berry for garnish; halve remaining berries and arrange evenly in bottom of a shallow 8-inch round broiler-proof dish.
4. Spoon cream mixture over berries.
5. Sprinkle remaining 1/4 cup brown sugar evenly over cream mixture.
6. Broil 4 to 5 inches from heat for 1 to 2 minutes or until sugar turns golden brown.
7. Slice reserved berry; arrange a top dessert.
8. Serve immediately.

Nutrition Facts (per serving)
Calories 187 Carbohydrates tdb
Protein 3 g Sodium 68 mg
Potassium 207 mg Phosphorus 59 mg

CORNBREAD MUFFINS

Ingredients:
Based on 12 servings per recipe.
1 cup all-purpose flour
1 cup cornmeal
1/2 teaspoon baking soda
1/4 cup granulated sugar

1/2 cup unsalted butter, softened
2 eggs
1/4 cup honey
1/2 cup buttermilk
1/2 cup no salt added canned corn

Directions:
1. Preheat oven to 400 degrees.
2. Use cooking oil spray to lightly grease a muffin pan.
3. In a large bowl, combine flour, cornmeal, baking soda and sugar.
4. Mix in butter using a pastry blender or mix in a food processor until butter is pea-sized.
5. In a separate bowl, beat eggs.
6. Mix in honey and buttermilk.
7. Pour egg mixture into the flour mixture stirring until just mixed.
8. Fold in the corn.
9. Spoon batter into muffin cups and bake for 20-25 minutes or until a toothpick inserted into the center of a muffin comes out clean.

Nutrition Facts (per serving)
Calories 203 Carbohydrates 28 g
Protein 4 g Sodium 79 mg
Potassium 89 mg Phosphorus 67 mg

PINEAPPLE PUDDING

Ingredients:
Yield: 12 servings Serving size: ½ cup
3 tablespoons all-purpose flour
½ cup sugar
1 large egg, whole
3 large eggs, divided
1 cup 2% milk

1 cup water
1 teaspoon vanilla extract
2 cups pineapple chunks, drained
¼ cup sugar
25-30 vanilla wafers

Directions:
Preheat oven to 425°F.
2. Combine flour, sugar, 1 whole egg and 3 egg yolks in top of a double boiler.
3. Stir in milk and water. Cook, uncovered over boiling water, stirring constantly, until thickened.
4. Remove from heat, and add vanilla extract.
5. Spread a small amount of the custard on the bottom of a 1 ½ quart casserole dish; top with half of the vanilla wafers, then half of the pineapple.
6. Continue with layers of custard, vanilla wafers, and pineapple, beginning and ending with custard.
7. Beat remaining egg whites with fork, egg beater, or hand mixer, add sugar. Beat until stiff peaks form.
8. Pile beaten egg whites on top of layered pudding. Bake for 5 minutes or until lightly browned.

Nutrition Facts (per serving)
Calories 209 Carbohydrates 38 g
Protein 4 g Sodium 80 mg Fat 5 g
Fiber 1 g Potassium 120 mg
Phosphorus 71 mg

EASTER EGG WREATH

Ingredients:
Based on 10-12 servings per recipe.

3/4 cup milk
1 package active dry yeast
1/4 cup butter or margarine
1/3 cup sugar
1 egg
3/4 teaspoon ground cardamom
2 3/4 - 3 cups flour
1/2 cup candied fruit (citron)
6 colored eggs (raw)

Directions:
1. Preheat oven to 375 degrees.
2. Warm 1/2 cup of milk in microwave about 1 minute.
3. Dissolve yeast in warm milk.
4. Cream together butter and sugar.
5. Beat in the egg, then add yeast mixture, remaining milk and cardamom.
6. Gradually mix in flour and candied fruit to make a moderately soft dough.
7. Turn out onto lightly-floured surface; knead till smooth and elastic, 5-8 minutes.
8. Place in lightly greased bowl, turning once to grease surface.
9. Cover; let rise till dough doubles in size, about 1 1/4 hours.
10. Punch down.
11. Turn out onto lightly floured surface and divide dough in thirds; form into balls.
12. Let rest for 10 minutes.
13. Roll each ball into a 16-inch long rope.
14. Line up the 3 ropes, 1 inch apart, on greased baking sheet.
15. Braid loosely, beginning in the middle and working towards the ends.
16. Pinch each end together and then form into a ring.
17. Fit colored eggs into folds of braid. They cook along with the bread!
18. Cover; let rise about 40 minutes, till dough has almost doubled in size.
19. Brush with a little milk.
20. Sprinkle with 1 Tbsp. sugar.
21. Bake for 20-25 minutes or until nicely browned.
22. Cool on wire rack

Nutrition Facts (per serving)
Calories 231 Carbohydrates 41 g
Protein 5 g Sodium 93 mg
Fiber 6 g Potassium 100 mg
Phosphorus 73 mg

PINEAPPLE POUND CAKE

Ingredients:
Yield: 24 servings Serving size: 1 slice (3 ½" x 4" x ¾")
For cake
3 cups sugar
1 ½ cups butter
6 whole eggs and 4 egg whites
1 teaspoon vanilla extract
3 cups all-purpose flour, sifted
1 10-ounce can crushed pineapple (drain and reserve juice)
For glaze
1 cup sugar
1 stick margarine
(½ cup) juice from pineapple

Directions:
1. Preheat oven to 350°F.
2. Beat together sugar and butter until smooth and creamy.
3. Add eggs and egg whites two at a time, mixing after each addition.

4. Add vanilla.
5. Add sifted flour and mix well.
6. Add drained, crushed pineapple.
7. Bake for 45 minutes to 1 hour.
8. In a medium saucepan, mix together ingredients for glaze.
Stir frequently. Bring to a boil, until desired thickness is reached. Pour over top of cake while hot.

Nutrition Facts (per serving)
Calories 288 Carbohydrates 47 g
Protein 2,5 g Sodium 93 mg Fat 9 g
Fiber 19 g Potassium 67 mg
Phosphorus 47 mg

8. Fold in whipped cream
9. Spread 1 ½ cups vanilla wafer crumbs in bottom of freezer tray or 10" x 6" x 1 ½" baking dish.
10. Spoon lemon mixture over crumbs.
11. Top with remaining vanilla wafer crumbs.
12. Freeze until firm, several hours or overnight.

Nutrition Facts (per serving)
Calories 205 Carbohydrates 23 g
Protein 3 g Sodium 97 mg Fat 7 g
Fiber 0 g Potassium 69 mg
Phosphorus 33 mg

FROZEN LEMON DESSERT

Ingredients:
Yield: 8 squares Serving size: 1 square
4 eggs, separated
⅔ cup sugar
¼ cup lemon juice
1 tablespoon lemon peel, grated
1 cup whipping cream, whipped
2 cups vanilla wafers (about 40), crushed
Directions:
1. Beat egg yolks until very thick.
2. Gradually beat in sugar, beating well after each addition.
3. Add lemon juice
and lemon peel; blend well.
4. Cook in double boiler over hot water stirring constantly until thick.
5. Remove from heat and allow to cool.
6. Beat egg whites until stiff peaks form.
7. Fold egg whites into cooled thickened mixture.

GINGERSNAP COOKIES

Ingredients:
Based on 3 dozen servings per recipe.
2 cups flour
1 tablespoon ginger, ground
2 teaspoons fresh ginger, finely grated
2 teaspoons baking soda
1 teaspoon cinnamon
3/4 cup shortening or unsalted butter
1 cup granulated sugar
1 egg
1/4 cup dark molasses
1/2 cup candied ginger, finely chopped
1/3 cup cinnamon sugar
Directions:
1. Preheat oven to 350 degrees.
2. Sift flour, ginger, baking soda, and cinnamon into mixing bowl.
3. Stir mixture to blend evenly.
4. Place the shortening into a different mixing bowl and beat until creamy.

5. Gradually beat in the granulated sugar.
6. Then beat in egg and molasses.
7. Sift 1/3 of flour mixture at a time into shortening mixture.
8. Stir to blend.
9. Mix together until soft dough forms.
10. Stir in candied ginger.
11. Pinch off small amounts of dough; roll into 1-inch diameter balls.
12. Roll each ball in cinnamon sugar and place two inches apart on an ungreased baking sheet.
13. Bake in preheated oven until the tops are rounded and slightly cracked, about 10 minutes.
14. Cool cookies on a wire rack.
15. Store cookies in an air-tight container or wrap dough in plastic wrap, freeze, and bake a few at a time later.

Nutrition Facts (per serving)
Calories 92 Carbohydrates 14 g
Protein 1 g Sodium 117 mg
Fiber 4 g Potassium 57 mg
Phosphorus 11 mg

ICE CREAM PUMPKIN PIE

Ingredients:
Based on 8 servings per recipe.
1 pint (2 cups) vanilla ice cream, softened
1 cup canned pumpkin
3/4 cup sugar
1/2 teaspoon ginger
1/2 teaspoon cinnamon
1/4 teaspoon nutmeg
1 cup whipped topping
1 9" baked pie shell

Directions:
1. Mix everything except pie shell in food processor until well blended.
2. Pour mixture into baked pie shell and freeze until firm.

Nutrition Facts (per serving)
Calories 275 Carbohydrates 42 g
Protein 3 g Sodium 118 mg
Potassium 90 mg Phosphorus 51 mg

NO-BAKE PEANUT BUTTER BALLS

Ingredients:
Based on 12 servings per recipe.
1/2 cup unsalted, unsweetened peanut butter
1 (8 ounce) package reduced fat cream cheese
1 1/4 cups graham cracker crumbs
1/4 cup mini chocolate chips
1 teaspoon vanilla
1/2 cup shredded coconut (optional)
Directions:
1. Mix all ingredients except coconut together, using an electric mixer until well blended.
2. Roll dough into one-inch balls.
3. Spread coconut evenly on a large plate.
4. Roll cookies in the coconut to lightly coat the outside (optional step).
5. Refrigerate for at least 1 hour or until the cookies become firm.
6. Store in the refrigerator for up to 1 week.
7. These cookies may also be frozen and thawed to enjoy late.

Nutrition Facts (per serving)
Calories 150 Carbohydrates 13 g
Protein 4 g Sodium 120 mg
Potassium 106 mg Phosphorus 65 mg

PUMPKIN SOUFFLE

Ingredients:
Yield: 1 pie (6 servings) Serving size: 1/6 portion
½ cup frozen apple juice concentrate (not diluted)
egg substitute equal to 2 whole eggs
1 12-ounce can pumpkin
1 cup whole milk
½ cup water
½ teaspoon vanilla extract
½ teaspoon ground nutmeg
½ teaspoon ground allspice
1 teaspoon ground cinnamon
½ cup grape nuts
½ teaspoon pumpkin pie spice (optional)

Directions:
1. Preheat oven to 400ºF.
2. Combine all ingredients except grape nuts in mixing bowl and stir well.
3. Spray 9" glass pie plate with cooking spray. Add mixture.
4. Sprinkle grape nuts on top.
5. Bake for 35 to 45 minutes or until knife inserted in center comes out clean.

Nutrition Facts (per serving)
Calories 129 Carbohydrates 26 g
Protein 5 g Sodium 120 mg Fat 1 g
Potassium 387 mg Phosphorus 112 mg

PINEAPPLE UPSIDE-DOWN CAKE

Ingredients:
Yield: 20 Squares Serving size: 1 square
2 sticks margarine
2 ½ cups sugar
1 teaspoons vanilla extract
4 eggs
4 egg whites
3 cups all-purpose flour, sifted
½ cup butter or margarine
1 16-ounce can crushed pineapple, drained
¾ cup brown sugar

Directions:
1. Preheat oven to 375°F.
2. Cream margarine until light and fluffy with electric mixer. Gradually add sugar; cream thoroughly.
3. Add vanilla extract, eggs and egg whites, two at a time.
4. Gradually add flour and mix well.
5. Melt ½ cup butter in a cake pan, preferably a sheet pan.
6. Spread pineapple evenly in pan; sprinkle brown sugar over pineapple.
7. Pour batter over pineapple. Bake for about 45 minutes.
8. When done, turn cake over onto a cake plate. Slice and serve.

Nutrition Facts (per serving)
Calories 301 Carbohydrates 52 g
Protein 4 g Sodium 123 mg Fat 9 g
Potassium 76 mg Phosphorus 26 mg

OLD FASHIONED POUND CAKE

Ingredients:
Yield: 24 servings Serving size: 1 slice (3 ½" x 4" x ¾")
2 cups butter or margarine
4 cups powdered sugar
2 tablespoons grated lemon rind
1 teaspoon lemon extract
6 eggs 3 ½ cups all-purpose flour, sifted

Directions:
1. Preheat oven to 350°F.
2. Using an electric mixer on medium speed, cream butter for 3 minutes, or until light and fluffy.
3. Gradually add sugar and rind; cream thoroughly.
4. Add lemon extract and eggs, one at a time, mixing well after each addition.
5. Gradually add flour; mix well.
6. Pour into greased and floured 10" tube pan or bundt pan.
7. Bake one hour and 20 minutes or until wooden pick inserted in center of cake comes out clean.
8. Remove from pan and cool.

Nutrition Facts (per serving)
Calories 279 Carbohydrates 34 g
Protein 10 g Sodium 127 mg Fat 11 g
Potassium 108 mg Phosphorus 139 mg

CREAM CHEESE POUND CAKE

Ingredients:
Yield: 40 cupcakes Serving size: 1 cupcake
For cake
3 sticks margarine or butter
8 ounces
cream cheese, softened
3 cups sugar
1 ½ teaspoon vanilla extract
4 large eggs
4 large egg whites
3 cups white cake flour, sifted
For frosting
2 16-ounce boxes powdered sugar
8 ounces cream cheese
1 stick margarine (½ cup)

Directions:
1. Preheat oven to 325°F.
2. Cream margarine, cream cheese, and sugar until light and fluffy.
3. Add vanilla, and beat well.
4. Add eggs, one at a time, and egg whites two at a time, beating well after each addition.
5. Stir in flour. Spoon mixture into a greased and floured muffin pan.
6. Bake for about 1 ½ hour.
7. Mix frosting and place on cooled cake.

Nutrition Facts (per serving)
Calories 285 Carbohydrates 46 g
Protein 3 g Sodium 133 mg Fat 3 g
Potassium 29 mg Phosphorus 16 mg

CHOCOLATE PIE SHELL

Ingredients:
Yield: 1 empty pie shell (6 servings)
Serving size: 1/6 portion
3 cups cocoa krispies, crushed
½ stick (4 tablespoons) butter cooking spray

Directions:
1. Place crushed cereal and melted butter in a bowl. Stir well.
2. Spray 9" pie pan with cooking spray.
3. Press mixture into pan.
4. Chill at least 30 minutes before filling.

Nutrition Facts (per serving)
Calories 126 Carbohydrates 18 g
Protein 2 g Sodium 135 mg Fat 6 g
Potassium 47 mg Phosphorus 24 mg

LEMON CHESS PIE

Ingredients:
Based on 8 servings per recipe.
1 9" single pie crust
1 1/2 cups sugar
6 tablespoons (3/4 stick) unsalted butter
3 tablespoons cornstarch
2 tablespoons lemon zest
4 large eggs
1/3 cup fresh lemon juice
1 cup whipped cream
to garnish fresh mint sprigs
Directions:
1. Preheat oven to 350 degrees.
2. Bake the pie crust until golden brown about 8 minutes or per package instructions.
3. Let cool.
4. Beat the sugar and butter in a large bowl until light and fluffy.
5. Add the cornstarch and lemon zest.
6. Add the eggs, one at a time, beating well after each addition.
7. Beat in the lemon juice and spoon the mixture into the pie shell.

8. Bake for 40-45 minutes, until the filling is set and the top is golden.
9. Cool.
10. Serve with a scoop of whipped cream and a small sprig of mint.

Nutrition Facts (per serving)
Calories 443 Carbohydrates 59 g
Protein 6 g Sodium 161 mg
Potassium 73 mg Phosphorus 69 mg

APPLE AND CREAM CHEESE TORTE

Ingredients:
Based on 10 servings per recipe.
1/2 cup unsalted butter, softened
3/4 cup sugar, divided in 1/4 cups
1 cup flour
8 ounces cream cheese, softened
1 egg
1 teaspoon vanilla
3-4 medium apples, thinly sliced
1/2 teaspoon cinnamon
Directions:
1. Preheat oven to 450 degrees.
2. In a medium bowl, cream butter and 1/4 cup of sugar.
3. Blend in flour.
4. Press into a spring form pan.
5. Beat cream cheese, 1/4 cup of sugar, egg, and vanilla until smooth.
6. Spread into the spring form pan.
7. Toss apples with remaining 1/4 cup of sugar and cinnamon.
8. Arrange apples over cheese filling.
9. Bake for 10 minutes.
10. Reduce oven temperature to 400

degrees and bake for an additional 25-30 minutes until filling is firm and the apples have softened.

Nutrition Facts (per serving)
Calories 298 Carbohydrates 36 g
Protein 4 g Sodium 176 mg
Potassium 102 mg Phosphorus 34 mg

WHIPPED CREAM POUND CAKE

Ingredients:
Yield: 30 slices Serving size: 1 slice
2 sticks margarine or butter, softened
3 cups sugar
6 eggs
3 cups cake flour (sift once before measuring)
½ pint whipping cream
1 teaspoon vanilla flavoring
Directions:
1. Preheat oven to 350°F.
2. Grease and flour tube pan.
3. All ingredients should be at room temperature.
4. Cream margarine and sugar together until fluffy.
5. Add eggs, one at a time, beating after each addition.
6. Gradually add flour and whipping cream, blending between each addition.
7. Beat well for 30 seconds; stir in vanilla flavoring.
8. Pour batter into tube pan; bake for 50-60 minutes.

Nutrition Facts (per serving)
Calories 249 Carbohydrates 35 g
Protein 8 g Sodium 192 mg Fat 9 g
Potassium 120 mg Phosphorus 24 mg

CHOCOLATE MINT CAKE

Ingredients:
Based on 12 servings per recipe.
2 cups all purpose flour
2 cups sugar
4 ounces unsweetened chocolate
2 teaspoons baking soda
1 teaspoon baking powder, low sodium
1 stick unsalted butter
1 cup water
1 cup heavy whipping cream
2 eggs
2 teaspoon peppermint extract
1 teaspoon apple cider vinegar
1 1/2 cups semisweet chocolate chip for frosting
1 1/2 cups sour cream for frosting
Directions:
1. Preheat oven to 375 degrees. To start, melt chocolate, butter, sugar, and water in a large saucepan over medium heat. Stirring occasionally until ingredients are well mixed. Transfer to a large mixing bowl and let cool
2. In a medium bowl, add flour, baking soda, and baking powder. In a small bowl, mix together cream and apple cider vinegar and set aside.
3. While the chocolate mixture is cooling, grease and flour two 9' round cake pans with butter. Adding a lining of parchment paper is suggested, as cake is very moist

and may stick to the pans.

4. Add the cream and vinegar mixture to the melted chocolate. Mix slightly then add eggs. Gently mix in dry ingredients, being careful to not over mix.

5. After all ingredients are well mixed, add the mint extract and gently whisk.

6. Pour cake batter into baking pans. Bake on center rack for 30-35 minutes or until toothpick inserted into the center comes out clean.

7. Let the cake cool for up to 30 minutes before removing from baking pans.

8. While cake is cooling, make the frosting. In a double boiler melt chocolate chips until smooth. After letting the chocolate cool for a couple minutes, slowly add sour cream until well mixed.

9. Once cake is completely cooled, frost and enjoy!

Nutrition Facts (per serving)
Calories 354 Carbohydrates 44 g
Protein 5 g Sodium 231 mg
Potassium 94 mg Phosphorus 82 mg

SUNNY ANGEL FOOD CAKE

Ingredients:
Based on 12 servings per recipe.
1 package angel food cake mix
1/2 of a 15 ounce can crushed pineapple (reserve juice)
1/2 of a 15 ounce can peaches, chopped (reserve juice)
1/2 pint heavy whipping cream
1/2 teaspoon vanilla extract
1/2 - 1 teaspoon lemon zest

1 tablespoon powdered or granulated sugar

Directions:
1. Mix cake per box directions using reserved juices in place of the water.
2. Add water if there is not enough juice.
3. Gently fold in canned fruit and bake per box directions.
4. Combine rest of ingredients and blend using an electric mixer until desired whipping cream consistancy is achieved.
5. Serve cake with whipping cream.

Nutrition Facts (per serving)
Calories 216 Carbohydrates 35 g
Protein 4 g Sodium 261 mg Fat 3 g
Potassium 123 mg Phosphorus 131 mg

CHOCOLATE MOCHA CHEESECAKE

Ingredients:
Based on 8 servings per recipe.
12 ounces chocolate wafer cookies
1/4 pound butter, unsalted
12 ounces chocolate chips
12 ounces cream cheese
1/4 cup sugar
6 eggs
1 cup whipping cream (unwhipped)
2 teaspoons vanilla
1/4 cup coffee liquer
Directions:
1. Preheat oven to 350 degree.
2. Crush wafer cookies.
3. Measure 3 cups of crumbs and cut in butter with a pastry blender.
4. Press into bottom and fill up to 3/4 of a 9" by 3" springform pan.

5. Refrigerate until firm.
6. Melt half the chocolate over simmering water. Let cool.
7. Beat cream cheese and sugar until light and fluffy; add eggs and beat well.
8. Add cream, vanilla, liquer and melted chocolate and blend well.
9. Remove crust from refrigerator and evenly add filling.
10. Place in oven for 1 hour, and then check if center is solid (does not jiggle when lightly shaken). Leave in if needed.
11. Melt remaining chocolate and pour over the top. Let cool to solidify before serving.

Nutrition Facts (per serving)
Calories 537 Carbohydrates 50 g
Protein 9 g Sodium 280 mg
Potassium 67 mg Phosphorus 52 mg

APPLE FILLED CREPES

Ingredients:
Based on 1 crepe servings per recipe.
4 egg yolks
2 whole eggs
1/2 cup sugar
1 cup flour
1/4 cup oil
2 cups milk
4 apples
1/2 cup brown sugar
1/2 teaspoon cinnamon
1/2 teaspoon nutmeg
1 stick or 1/2 cup unsalted butter
Directions:
1. Mix egg yolks, whole eggs, sugar, flour, oil, and milk until the batter is free of lumps.
2. Heat a small non-stick skillet over medium heat.
3. Spray pan with cooking spray.
4. Using a 2 ounce ladle or 1/4 cup, spoon 1 scoop of batter into the pan, then swirl the pan to spread the crepe batter thinly on the bottom of the pan.
5. Cook for about 20 seconds, then flip the crepe (with the aid of a rubber spatula) and cook for about 10 seconds. filling.
6. Peel, core, and slice apples each into 12 slices.
7. Heat a medium saute pan.
8. Melt butter, then add brown sugar.
9. Toss in the apples, cinnamon, and nutmeg.
10. Cook apples until tender but not mushy. Set aside to cool.
11. Assembling the Crepes: Fill the middle of each crepe about with about 2 tablespoons of apple filling.
12. Roll into a log.
Note: Crepes can be made the day before or hours in advance, just cover with plastic wrap and store in the refrigerator. When ready to eat microwave crepes for a few seconds

Nutrition Facts (per serving)
Calories 315 Carbohydrates 40 g
Protein 5 g Sodium 356 mg
Potassium 160 mg Phosphorus 103 mg

ZUCCHINI PROV

Ingredients: 2 potatoes
5 large zucchini
2 red bell pepper
2 tomatoes
1/2 cup green onions, chopped
1/2 teaspoon basil
1 cup celery, chopped
2 tablespoons oil

Directions:
1. Dice potatoes into 1/2 inch pieces and cut zucchini into 1 inch chunks.
2. Slice bell peppers.
3. If using whole tomatoes, quarter and slice though again.
4. In a large pan, saute onions, basil, and celery in oil.
5. Add tomatoes, zucchini and potatoes.
6. Stir gently, then cover and steam until tender.

Nutrition Facts (per serving)
Calories 144 Carbohydrates 21 g
Protein 4 g Sodium 38 mg
Potassium 988 mg Phosphorus 131 mg

ROASTED PAPRIKA-LACED CAULIFLOWER

Ingredients:
Based on 6-8 servings per recipe.
1 head (about 1/2 cup per person) cauliflower, cut into florets
2 tablespoons olive oil
Juice of 1/2 lemon, about 2 tablespoons
1 teaspoon paprika
Black pepper to taste

Directions:
1. Preheat oven to 400 degrees F.
2. In a large bowl or large Ziploc bag, mix the cauliflower, olive oil, and lemon juice. Toss or shake until cauliflower is well coated.
3. Add paprika and black pepper, coat or shake well.
4. Place cauliflower in a shallow roasting pan or cookie sheet and cook for 25-40 minutes until the cauliflower is tender and lightly browned.

Nutrition Facts (per serving)
Calories 78 Carbohydrates 8 g
Protein 3 g Sodium 43 mg Fat 5 g
Potassium 429 mg Phosphorus 62 mg

SEASONED PORK CHOPS

Ingredients:
Yield: 4 chops Serving size: 1 chop (3-ounces)
2 tablespoons vegetable oil
¼ cup all-purpose flour
1 teaspoon black pepper
½ teaspoon sage
½ teaspoon thyme
4 4-ounce lean pork chops (fat removed)

Directions:
1. Preheat oven to 350ºF.
2. Grease baking pan with vegetable oil.
3. Mix flour, black pepper, thyme and sage.
4. Dredge pork chops in flour mixture and arrange in baking pan.

5. Place in oven and let brown on both sides about 40 minutes or until tender.
6. Remove from oven. Serve hot.

Nutrition Facts (per serving)
Calories 434 Carbohydrates 12 g
Protein 19 g Sodium 60 mg Fat 34 g
Potassium 332 mg Phosphorus 199 mg

OVEN BLASTED VEGETABLES

Ingredients:
Based on 4-6 servings per recipe.
1 yukon gold potato
3/4 cup carrots
1 onion
1 yam
1 beet
2 tablespoons olive oil
1/4 cup fruit vinegar to taste parmesan cheese
Directions:
1. Cut vegetables into equal sized pieces, either coin shaped or lengthwise.
2. In a 500 degree oven, heat oil in a flat metal pan for 2 minutes.
3. Add cubed potatoes, carrots, and onion, cook 10 minutes.
4. Stir, cook 5 more minutes, add yam and beets, cook 20 minutes, stirring every 10 minutes.
5. Remove from heat, sprinkle with vinegar & grated parmesan and serve.

Nutrition Facts (per serving)
Calories 247 Carbohydrates 40 g
Protein 5 g Sodium 62 mg
Potassium 243 mg Phosphorus 67 mg

ITALIAN MEATBALLS

Ingredients:
Based on 12 (2 meatballs each) servings per recipe.
1.5 pounds ground beef
2 large eggs, beaten
1/2 cup dry oatmeal flakes
3 tablespoons parmesan cheese
1/2 tablespoon olive oil
1/2 tablespoon garlic powder
1 teaspoon dried oregano
1/2 cup onion, chopped
1/2 teaspoon black pepper
Directions:
1. Preheat oven to 375 degrees.
2. Combine all ingredients in a large bowl and mix together.
3. Roll into 1" balls and place on a baking sheet.
4. Bake for 10 to 15 minutes, until meatballs are cooked through.
5. To serve, place meatballs in a warming dish or crock pot on low heat setting. Serve with 2 teaspoons sauce on the side.

Nutrition Facts (per serving)
Calories 163 Carbohydrates 4 g
Protein 13 g Sodium 72 mg
Potassium 199 mg Phosphorus 125 mg

CRISPY OVEN FRIED CHICKEN

Ingredients:
Yield: 8 servings (or 8 pieces) Serving size: 3 or 4-ounces
2 ½ pound fryer (cut as desired)
1 tablespoon lemon juice

1 cup all-purpose flour
1 teaspoon black pepper
1 cup corn flakes, crushed
¼ teaspoon poultry seasoning
4 tablespoons vegetable oil

Directions:
1. Preheat oven to 400ºF.
2. Wash chicken parts thoroughly and pat dry; rub with lemon juice.
3. In a small bag, combine flour, black pepper, corn flakes, and poultry seasoning. Shake well.
4. In a shallow baking pan (about 1" deep), grease with vegetable oil.
5. Place chicken in bag of ingredients, using the largest pieces first. Shake well.
6. Arrange coated chicken in pan.
7. Brown in oven 20-30 minutes on each side.

Nutrition Facts (per serving)
Calories 280 Carbohydrates 15 g
Protein 15 g Sodium 74 mg
Potassium 150 mg Phosphorus 120 mg

CROCK POT WHITE CHICKEN CHILI

Ingredients:
Based on 12-14 servings per recipe.
1 cup dried Great Northern beans
1 cup dried black eyed peas
1 cup dried lima beans
1/2 cup dried small lima beans
8 cups water
2 medium onions, diced
3 tablespoons minced garlic
2 pounds chicken breast, diced

1-2 jalapeño chili peppers, diced
2 tablespoons vegetable oil or canola
2 cups frozen corn
2 teaspoons cumin
2 teaspoons oregano
1 teaspoon black pepper
1/2 teaspoon cayenne pepper
2 cups sour cream

Directions:
1. Rinse and sort the dried beans.
2. Place beans in Crock-Pot (slow cooker) with water.
3. Set temperature to low.
4. Meanwhile, sauté onions, garlic, diced chicken, and jalapeños in vegetable or canola oil in a skillet for about 10 minutes, until lightly browned.
5. Add to the Crock-Pot.
6. Add corn and spices to mixture.
7. Let cook 9-11 hours, or overnight.
8. Before serving, stir in the sour cream.

Nutrition Facts (per serving)
Calories 306 Carbohydrates 32 g
Protein 25 g Sodium 74 mg Fat 12 g
Potassium 845 mg Phosphorus 321 mg

FAST ROAST CHICKEN WITH LEMON & HERBS

Ingredients:
Based on 4-6 (3 ounce servings) servings per recipe.
1 (4-5 pound) whole chicken, fresh or thawed
2 tablespoons unsalted butter, softened
2 1/2 tablespoons chopped fresh herbs (sage, thyme, etc)

2 cloves garlic, peeled and crushed
1 small lemon, thinly sliced
1 tablespoon olive oil
Directions:
1. Preheat oven to 450 degrees.
2. Place the chicken in a roasting pan.
3. Mix the butter, herbs and garlic together in a small bowl.
4. Place the herbed butter inside the body cavity of the chicken, along with the lemon slices.
5. Rub the olive oil over the skin of the bird.
6. Roast for 15 minutes per pound, or until internal temperature reaches 165 degrees.
7. Drain the buttery juices and slices of lemon and pour over chicken.
8. Let chicken rest for 20 minutes before carving.

Nutrition Facts (per serving)
Calories 251 Carbohydrates 0 g
Protein 19 g Sodium 77 mg
Potassium 222 mg Phosphorus 188 mg

CHILI RICE WITH BEEF

Ingredients:
Yield: 4 servings Serving size: 1 cup
2 tablespoons vegetable oil
1 pound
lean ground beef
1 cup onion, chopped
2 cups rice, cooked
1 ½ teaspoons chili con carne seasoning powder
⅛ teaspoon black pepper

½ teaspoon sage
Directions:
1. Heat oil; add beef and onion. Cook, stirring occasionally until browned.
2. Add rice and seasonings.Mix together.
3. Remove from heat. Cover and let stand 10-14 minutes.

Nutrition Facts (per serving)
Calories 360 Carbohydrates 26 g
Protein 23 g Sodium 78 mg Fat 14 g
Potassium 427 mg Phosphorus 233 mg

STUFFED ZUCCHINI

Ingredients:
Based on 6 servings per recipe.
1 very large zucchini or 3-5 small zucchini
1 12 oz can low sodium diced tomatoes
¼ cup mixed fresh herbs, (any combination of oregano, thyme, sage) or 2 tablespoons dried Italian seasoning
¼ cup fresh flat leaf parsley, chopped fine
¼ teaspoon black pepper
1 onion, diced fine
6-8 cloves whole fresh garlic, peeled and smashed
2-3 tablespoons olive oil
¼ cup Parmesan cheese, shaved
Directions:
1. Preheat oven to 350 degrees.
2. If using a large zucchini, slice it in half lengthwise. Scoop out the inside and cube, discarding any parts with very large seeds. If using small zucchini, peel

and cube.

3. In a medium sauce pan, add tomatoes, fresh herbs, parsley, and pepper. Simmer.

4. Meanwhile, in a fry pan, sauté onion and garlic in olive oil. Add cubed zucchini and sauté until golden on edges. Add tomato sauce and mix in.

5. If using large zucchini, place halves, cut side up, in greased baking pan. Fill with zucchini and tomato mixture. If using small zucchini, fill greased baking dish.

6. Top with large shavings of Parmesan.

7. Bake in oven about 15 minutes, serve

Nutrition Facts (per serving)
Calories 117 Carbohydrates 13 g
Protein 4 g Sodium 86 mg
Potassium 578 mg Phosphorus 109 mg

FRUIT VINEGAR CHICKEN

Ingredients:
Based on 6 servings per recipe.
2 pounds chicken
1/2 cup fruit or berry vinegar
1/4 cup oil
1/4 cup orange juice
1/2 teaspoon marjoram
1/2 teaspoon basil
1/2 teaspoon tarragon
Directions:
1. Preheat oven to 350 degrees.
2. Combine all ingredients in a large zip lock bag.
3. Marinade for 15-20 minutes in the refrigerator.

4. Remove chicken from bag, and place in a baking dish.

5. Bake for about 30 minutes or until chicken reaches an internal temperature of 165 degrees.

Nutrition Facts (per serving)
Calories 413 Carbohydrates 3 g
Protein 28 g Sodium 106 mg
Potassium 335 mg Phosphorus 227 mg

GRILLED LEMON CHICKEN KEBABS

Ingredients:
Based on 2 servings per recipe.
4 pieces boneless, skinless chicken thighs
2 lemons
3 tablespoons olive oil
1 clove garlic, peeled and crushed
1 tablespoon chopped fresh herbs(sage thyme, etc)
2 bay leaves, torn in half
1 teaspoon white wine vinegar
Directions:
1. Chop each thigh into chunky pieces and place in a bowl.
2. Grate 1 teaspoon lemon zest and juice the remaining whole lemon.
3. Add to the chicken along with the oil, garlic, herbs and vinegar.
4. Cover and marinate for at least 3 hours, or overnight.
5. Slice the other lemon into 4 thick slices, then cut each slice into 4 pieces.
6. On a wooden skewer, alternate the lemon slices and the chicken pieces,

packing as tight as possible, finishing off with a lemon piece.

7. Repeat for each skewer.

8. Grill until done, about 10 minutes each side, in the oven, barbecue or countertop-type grill.

Nutrition Facts (per serving)
Calories 362 Carbohydrates 6 g
Protein 27 g Sodium 119 mg
Potassium 404 mg Phosphorus 238 mg

HONEY HERB GLAZED TURKEY

Ingredients:
Based on 6-8 servings per recipe.
10-12 pounds whole turkey
1 onion, cut into wedges
2 celery stalks, whole
1 lemon, cut into chunks
1/3 cup olive oil
1/2 cup unsalted butter
2 tablespoons fresh sage leaves
1/3 cup fresh thyme stripped from stems (about 14 stems)
2 fresh bay leaves
2 teaspoons celery seed
1/4 cup honey
2 teaspoons lemon juice

Directions:
1. Heat oven to 350 degrees.
2. Remove neck and giblets from turkey.
3. Fill bird with onion, celery and lemon.
4. Rub skin with olive oil.
5. Put on 2 sheets of aluminum foil.
6. Cover top of bird with seperate sheet of foil, which you will remove later.
7. Seal the edges of the foil and put on a rack and roast in the oven.

8. While turkey is cooking, melt butter, chop sage and thyme leaves finely.

9. Add bay leaves, chopped herbs, and honey to butter.

10. Simmer 10 minutes, until butter is lightly browned, then remove the bay leaves.

11. When the turkey reaches 145-155 degrees, raise oven temperature to 500 degrees, remove top foil and baste turkey with honey herb mixture, every 5-10 minutes or so.

12. Using a thermometer, when the turkey reaches 160 degrees remove from oven, tent with foil and let rest 30 minutes before carving.

Nutrition Facts (per serving)
Calories 412 Carbohydrates 7 g
Protein 49 g Sodium 119 mg
Potassium 526 mg Phosphorus 357 mg

TEXAS HASH

Ingredients: Based on 8 (1 cup each) servings per recipe.
1 1/2 pounds (24 ounces) ground turkey
1 green bell pepper, chopped
1 onion, chopped
2 tablespoons chili powder
1/2 cup rice
1 (14.5 ounce) can no salt added tomatoes (do not drain)

Directions:
1. Preheat oven to 350 degrees.
2. Cook turkey, green peppers, and onion in a skillet.
3. When the turkey is almost cooked

and vegetables are tender (about 10-15 minutes), add chili powder, rice and tomatoes.

4. Pour mixture into a medium casserole dish and cover with foil.

5. Bake in oven for 40 minutes or 60 minutes if using brown rice.

Nutrition Facts (per serving)
Calories 207 Carbohydrates 15 g
Protein 17 g Sodium 134 mg Fat 2 g
Potassium 427 mg Phosphorus 177 mg

PARSLIED ONIONS AND PINTO BEANS

Ingredients:
Based on 8-12 servings per recipe.
1 cup Italian parsley, flat-leafed
1 cup curly parsley
1/2 cup fresh dill
1 large lemon
2 cups low salt chicken broth
2 tablespoons butter
1 tablespoon oil
6 cups onions, sliced
1/2 teaspoon curry powder
4 cups pinto beans, low sodium
to taste pepper

Directions:
1. Wash and dry the parsley and dill.
2. Remove any thick stems and chop into 1/2 – 1 inch pieces; set aside.
3. Halve the lemon and squeeze the juice; set aside.
4. Put the halved lemon and broth in a small saucepan.
5. Bring the broth to a boil, lower heat, and simmer, covered.

6. In a large saucepan, heat the butter and oil and cook the onions until wilted and golden.
7. Stir in the curry powder, parsley, and dill.
8. Add the broth and lemon halves.
9. Cook slowly to tenderize the parsley and slightly reduce the broth. (If you cover the pan, the parsley loses some of its brilliant color.)
10. Stir in the beans and the lemon juice and heat through.
11. Remove lemon halves.
12. Season with pepper.

Nutrition Facts (per serving)
Calories 458 Carbohydrates 78 g
Protein 26 g Sodium 140 mg
Potassium 207 mg Phosphorus 432 mg

HERB BREADED CHICKEN

Ingredients:
Based on 4 servings per recipe.
1/4 teaspoon basil
1/4 teaspoon thyme
1/4 teaspoon oregano
1/4 teaspoon tarragon
1/4 teaspoon paprika
1/4 teaspoon fresh ground black pepper
1 1/2 slices whole wheat bread
1 pound boneless chicken breasts or 1 1/2 pounds "bone in" chicken

Directions:
1. Preheat oven to 400 degrees.
2. Combine herbs and spices in blender or food processor with bread.

3. Mix well.
4. Dip chicken in herb mixture.
5. Bake in a single layer for 20 minutes (boneless chicken) or 50 minutes (bone-in).

Nutrition Facts (per serving)
Calories 172 Carbohydrates 7 g
Protein 27 g Sodium 180 mg Fiber 3 g
Potassium 444 mg Phosphorus 249 mg

PANCIT GUISADO

Ingredients:
Based on 6 servings per recipe.
8 ounces rice stick noodles (bihon)
1/4 cup vegetable oil
3 cloves garlic, minced
1/2 medium onion, chopped
1 pound chicken breast or pork, boiled & sliced
1 1/2 cups shredded green cabbage
1 large carrot, peeled & cut like matchsticks
1 tablespoon reduced sodium soy sauce
1 cup low sodium chicken broth
1 stalk celery, sliced
2 green onions, chopped
1 lemon (optional)
Directions:
1. Soak rice noodles in warm water for 5 minutes, drain and set aside.
2. Heat oil in a large skillet or wok over medium heat.
3. Add garlic and onion and saute for 5 minutes.
4. Add sliced meat, cabbage, and carrots.
5. Stir- fry for 3 minutes.
6. Add reduced sodium soy sauce,

chicken broth, and celery.
7. Simmer for 3 minutes.
8. Add soaked rice noodles to broth and simmer for 3 minutes.
9. Top noodles with meat and vegetable mixture, garnish with green onions and flavor with fresh squeezed lemon juice, if desired.

Nutrition Facts (per serving)
Calories 287 Carbohydrates 39 g
Protein 19 g Sodium 194 mg
Potassium 391 mg Phosphorus 183 mg

MASTER GROUND BEEF MIX

Ingredients:
Based on 8 servings per recipe.
2 pounds ground beef
1 cup diced onion
3 tablespoons Worcestershire sauce
1 teaspoon Italian seasoning
1 teaspoon garlic powder
1/4 teaspoon pepper
4 slices white bread, cubed
1/2 cup milk
Directions:
1. In a large fry pan, on the stove top, mix all ingredients.
2. Cook, stirring occasionally, until meat is no longer red.
3. Remove meat from heat, drain excess liquid.
4. Let cool in the refrigerator.
5. Portion 1 cup meat in to freeze containers or freezer weight bags.
6. Freeze for later use in tacos, Shepard's pie, nachos, stroganoff, goulash, soups,

or casseroles.
7. Keeps for 3 months in the freeze

Nutrition Facts (per serving)
Calories 331 Carbohydrates 13 g
Protein 32 g Sodium 215 mg
Potassium 482 mg Phosphorus 256 mg

TEXAS-STYLE CHILI

Ingredients:
Based on 6 servings per recipe.
1 pound lean ground beef
1 large onion
1 (8 ounce) can tomato sauce (unsalted if possible)
2 cups water
1 (4 ounce) can green chili pepper, chopped
1 orange or red bell pepper, chopped
2 tablespoons chili powder
1 tablespoon garlic powder
1/4 teaspoon ground cumin
1/2 teaspoon dried oregano
1/2 teaspoon dried thyme
1 teaspoon dried basil
1/4 teaspoon cajun seasoning
Directions:
1. In a large pot, cook beef over medium heat until browned.
2. Stir in onion and cook until soft.
3. Stir in tomato sauce, 2 cups water, green chilis, bell pepper, and spices.
4. Bring to a boil then reduce heat to medium-low and simmer for at least one hour.

Nutrition Facts (per serving)
Calories 225 Carbohydrates 10 g
Protein 21 g Sodium 218 mg
Potassium 490 mg Phosphorus 168 mg

STIR-FRY PEPPER STEAK

Ingredients:
Based on 4 servings per recipe.
2 tablespoons cooking sherry or unseasond rice vinegar
1 tablespoon Homemade Low-Sodium Soy Sauce (our recipes)
1 teaspoon cornstarch
1 pound lean flank steak or chuck steak cut into thin strips
1-2 bell peppers sliced into strips
1 medium onion, sliced
1 clove garlic, crushed
4 plum tomatoes, cut into 6ths
2 cups broccoli
2 tablespoons vegetable oil, divided
2 tablespoons grated fresh ginger
1/2 teaspoon sugar
1/4 cup water
For Sauce: 1 tablespoon cornstarch
2 tablespoons water
2 tablespoons (our) Homemade Low-Sodium Soy Sauce
Directions:
1. Combine sherry or rice vinegar with Homemade Low-Sodium Soy Sauce, cornstarch and beef.
2. Marinate for 15 minutes.
3. While marinating, cut up peppers, onions, garlic, and tomatoes.
4. Heat 1 tablespoon oil until hot.
5. Fry onion & peppers for one minute.

6. Add garlic, tomatoes, sugar, ginger and water.

7. Stir fry for another minute.

8. Remove from pan and set aside.

9. Combine cornstarch, water, and soy sauce, set aside.

10. Heat one tablespoon oil until hot: stir fry marinated beef until meat changes color.

11. Add vegetables and thicken with cornstarch mixture.

12. Serve hot over noodles or rice.

Nutrition Facts (per serving)
Calories 296 Carbohydrates 18 g
Protein 26 g Sodium 220 mg
Potassium 624 mg Phosphorus 275 mg

PAELLA

Ingredients:
Based on 6-8 servings per recipe.
1 tablespoon olive oil
1/2 pound Italian sausage
1/2 pound chicken breast, diced
1-2 garlic cloves, pressed
2 cups uncooked short grain rice
1 cup yellow onion, chopped
1 1/2 cups low sodium chicken broth
2 jars roasted red peppers, pureed
1/2 teaspoon paprika
1/2 teaspoon Tabasco sauce
10 strands or 1/8 teaspoon saffron
1/2 pound shrimp, uncooked, shelled, deveined
1/2 cup each red & green peppers, sliced in strips
1/2 cup frozen green peas
Directions:

1. Heat olive oil in large pan and saute sausage, chicken, and garlic until meat is browned.

2. Remove meats and set aside.

3. Add rice and onion to pan and saute until onion is translucent and rice is golden brown.

4. Add meat back to pan with broth and pureed red bell peppers.

5. Add paprika, Tabasco, and saffron.

6. Bring to a boil; reduce heat to low, and simmer covered for 10 minutes.

7. Stir in shrimp, bell peppers, and peas.

8. Cover and cook 10 minutes.

Nutrition Facts (per serving)
Calories 223 Carbohydrates 25 g
Protein 20 g Sodium 257 mg
Potassium 330 mg Phosphorus 201 mg

CHICKEN LASAGNA WITH WHITE SAUCE

Ingredients:
Based on 6 servings per recipe.
6 ounces chicken (breast or thigh)
12 ounces low sodium chicken broth
1/4 cup olive oil
1 large onion, diced
1 tablespoon oregano
1/4 teaspoon black pepper
1/4 cup white wine (optional)
1/2 cup mushrooms, thick sliced
3 tablespoons flour
6 ounces cream cheese
1 1/2 cups Mocha Mix (or any non-dairy creamer)
1/4-1/2 teaspoon nutmeg

1/2 cup fresh parmesan cheese, grated
1 1/2 zucchini, sliced into little moons
1 package no boil lasagna noodles
Directions:
1. Pre-heat oven to 375 degrees.
2. Place chicken and broth in small pot and bring to boil, reduce heat to simmer until chicken is white and fully cooked. Chicken will cook faster if cut into pieces.
3. Meanwhile, in a large saute pan, over medium heat, add olive oil, onion, oregano, and black pepper and saute for 5 minutes or until onion begins to soften.
4. If using wine, add to pan and allow to evaporate.
5. Add mushrooms.
6. Sprinkle flour evenly over pan, stirring to distribute flavors. Ingredients in pan should look clumpy.
7. Allow this to cook for a few minutes (~3 minutes).
8. Break up cream cheese and add to pan, stirring once again until melted and evenly distributed. (~2 minutes)
9. Slowly add Mocha mix to the pan, stirring once again.
10. Ingredients should be thickening up and not be clumpy. If it's still clumpy, keep stirring to break them up.
11. Add nutmeg.
12. Stir in parmesan cheese and keep stirring as it cooks for another 5 minutes, the sauce should also be thickening up.
13. Remove chicken from pot (save the broth) and using two forks, shred chicken apart, trying to keep pieces even.
14. Set aside.
15. Stir in 1/2 cup of leftover broth into cream mixture to thin it out, stirring occasioanlly for 2 minutes.

16. Place lasagna sheets into pan, top with 1/3 of the sauce, then 1/2 the chicken, and 1/2 of the zucchini pieces (evenly spread on top); repeat layers again, topping it off with the remaining sauce.
17. Cover in foil and place in oven for 30 minutes, and remove foil for last few minutes until desired crispiness.

RAIN CITY STUFFED SHELLS

Ingredients:
Based on 6 servings per recipe.
1 package large pasta shells or manicotti tubes
1 half carton (about 2 cups) ricotta cheese
2 large eggs, beaten
1 bunch baby spinach
1/2 cup fresh basil, chopped
large can low sodium tomato sauce
enough grated parmesan cheese to garnish
Directions:
1. Heat oven to 350 degrees.
2. Start large pot of boiling water for pasta.
3. Add shells and cook only about 4-5 minutes (you want them stiff enough to hold their shape).
4. Meanwhile, put the baby spinach in a bowl and microwave about 2-3 minutes (should be wilted), then coarsley chop.
5. Mix ricotta, cooked spinach, basil, and eggs together.
6. Rinse pasta in cold water.
7. Using a spoon, fill the shells.

8. Put 1/2 the sauce on the bottom of a greased casserole dish, setting shells filled side up.
9. Drizzle top with remaining sauce, sprinkle with parmesan and bake uncovered about 30 minutes.

Nutrition Facts (per serving)
Calories 426 Carbohydrates 66 g
Protein 19 g Sodium 277 mg
Potassium 191 mg Phosphorus 270 mg

QUICK FETTUCCINE

Ingredients:
Based on 6 servings per recipe.
1/2 - 2/3 cup boiling water
1 package penne pasta
2-3 cloves garlic, minced
1 teaspoon canola oil
1 cup meat, fish, shrimp of choice
1-2 cups veggies (asparagus, broccoli, peas)
1 (8 ounce) package Neufchatel or cream cheese
1/2 cup fresh parmesan cheese, grated
1/4 cup fresh parsley
1/4 cup fresh basil
Directions:
1. Start boiling pasta water.
2. Once water is boiling, remove about 2/3 cup boiling water and add pasta.
3. While waiting for water to boil, sauté garlic in oil in frying pan.
4. If adding meat or veggies, sauté until done with garlic.
5. In food processor or blender, mix cheeses and fresh herbs and 1/2 cup of

the hot water.
6. If sauce is too thick, add more water.
7. Pour into fry pan over sautéed garlic and veggies/meat if you choose.
8. Pour over pasta.

Nutrition Facts (per serving)
Calories 304 Carbohydrates 32 g
Protein 18 g Sodium 285 mg
Potassium 216 mg Phosphorus 121 mg

SPICY HONEY MUSTARD CHICKEN

Ingredients:
Based on 6 servings per recipe.
3 tablespoons dijon mustard
3 tablespoons honey
2 tablespoons Mrs. Dash Extra Spicy Seasoning
1 1/2 pounds chicken breast, cut into strips
1 tablespoon vegetable or olive oil
Directions:
1. Mix mustard, honey and Mrs. Dash in a large bowl, reserve 1-2 tablespoons for dipping if you like.
2. Add chicken and coat thoroughly with mustard mixture.
3. Heat skillet with oil and place over medium-high heat.
4. Add chicken to the pan and cook until golden brown and completely cooked through, about 3-4 minutes per side.
5. For a little added spice try serving with our Coleslaw with a Kick

Nutrition Facts (per serving)
Calories 180 Carbohydrates 9 g
Protein 25 g Sodium 287 mg
Potassium 237 mg Phosphorus 183 mg

TACO POCKETS

Ingredients:
Based on 4 servings per recipe.
8 ounces cooked shredded chicken
1/4 cup diced purple onion
2 ounces shredded cheddar cheese
2 pita pocket breads (6" in diameter)
1 tablespoon lemon juice
1 medium chopped tomato
2 tablespoons French salad dressing
1 tablespoon taco sauce
1 cup shredded lettuce
Directions:
1. In a bowl, combine chicken, onion, and cheese.
2. Cut pita in half.
3. Spoon one quarter of mixture into each pita half.
4. Wrap in foil or parchment paper to hold together. Refrigerate until serving.
5. Mix dressing and taco sauce in a small bowl.
6. To serve, drizzle 2 tablespoons of sauce over chicken filling on sandwich and top with lettuce. Keeps 3 days refrigerated.

Nutrition Facts (per serving)
Calories 277 Carbohydrates 22 g
Protein 23 g Sodium 367 mg
Potassium 397 mg Phosphorus 194 mg

JAMMIN' JAMBALAYA

Ingredients:
Based on 6 servings per recipe.
2 teaspoons olive oil
1/2 pound jumbo shrimp, cooked, tails removed
7 ounces smoked turkey sausage, sliced
1/2 large yellow onion, chopped
1 large red bell pepper, chopped
3 cups collard greens, chopped
2 garlic cloves, minced
1/4 teaspoon cayenne pepper
1/8 teaspoon white pepper
1/4 teaspoon black pepper
1/2 teaspoon dry thyme or 1-2 teaspoons fresh thyme
1/2 teaspoon oregano
2 bay leaves
1/4 teaspoon allspice
1/2 cup rice (white or brown)
1 2/3 cups chicken broth
Directions:
Heat olive oil in a large skillet over medium-high heat.
1. Add shrimp, turkey sausage, onion, bell pepper, collards and garlic.
2. Cook for 10 minutes, stirring occasionally.
3. Add remaining ingredients and bring to a boil.
4. Cover, reduce heat to medium-low and simmer for 20 minutes or until rice is tender. (35-40 if using brown rice).

Nutrition Facts (per serving)
Calories 200 Carbohydrates 19 g
Protein 16 g Sodium 400 mg
Potassium 314 mg Phosphorus 170 mg

PUFFY CHILI RELLENOS CASSEROLE

Ingredients:
Based on 8 servings per recipe.
6 ounces cheddar cheese, shredded
6 ounces jack cheese, shredded
1 cup ricotta cheese
8 fresh padillia peppers, whole
8 large eggs
2/3 cup milk
1 cup flour
1 teaspoon baking powder, low sodium

Directions:
1. Preheat oven to 350 degrees.
2. Roast peppers and remove skins. See roasting instructions below.
3. Put cheese and ricotta in peppers and arrange in a greased 9×13 pan.
4. In blender or food processor beat eggs, milk, flour, and baking powder until smooth.
5. Pour evenly over peppers.
6. Bake for 30-40 minutes.
7. Serve hot.

Nutrition Facts (per serving)
Calories 273 Carbohydrates 22 g
Protein 24 g Sodium 420 mg Fat 2 g
Potassium 388 mg Phosphorus 325 mg

TUNA LOAF

Ingredients:
Based on 4 servings per recipe.
12 ounces Tuna or Salmon, water packed
2 eggs, beaten

1 cup milk
2 tablespoons green pepper, chopped
1 tablespoon onion, chopped
1/8 teaspoon pepper
1/4 teaspoon Worcestershire sauce

Directions:
1. Preheat oven to 350 degrees.
2. Mix all ingredients in a large bowl.
3. Pour into greased loaf pan (or form patties and pan fry).
4. Bake for 35 minutes.
5. Serve hot with our Sour Cream Dill Sauce recipe

Nutrition Facts (per serving)
Calories 158 Carbohydrates 4 g
Protein 26 g Sodium 456 mg
Potassium 141 mg Phosphorus 109 mg

CHICKEN WITH CORNBREAD STUFFING

Ingredients:
Based on 4 servings per recipe.
1 tablespoon fresh parsley
2 tablespoons + 1 1/2 teaspoons Mrs. Dash Original Blend, divided
1 tablespoon Mrs. Dash Chicken Grilling Blend
4 (4 ounce) pieces boneless, skinless chicken breast halves
1 tablespoon unsalted butter
1 cup celery, chopped
1/2 cup onion, chopped
2 teaspoons ground sage
2 cups (about 7 ounces) cornbread, coarsely crumbled
2 cups unseasoned croutons

1 cup fat-free low sodium chicken broth
Directions:
1. Chop parsley.
2. Combine 1 tablespoon Mrs. Dash® Original Blend, Mrs. Dash® Chicken Grilling Blend™, parsley, mix lightly.
3. Coat chicken breasts on both sides with seasoning blend mixture.
4. Spray large non-stick skillet with non-stick cooking spray.
5. Heat skillet over medium heat until hot.
6. Add chicken breasts to skillet, cook 3 to 5 minutes on each side or until lightly brown.
7. Remove chicken breasts from skillet, set aside.
8. Preheat oven to 350 degrees.
9. Melt butter in skillet over low heat.
10. Add celery, onion, 1 tablespoon + 1 1/2 teaspoons Mrs. Dash® Original Blend, sage, mixing to blend.
11. Cook over medium heat 5 to 7 minutes or until vegetables are tender.
12. Remove from heat.
13. Combine cornbread crumbs and croutons in mixing bowl.
14. Add vegetable mixture and broth, mixing to blend.
15. Spoon dressing mixture to large baking dish lightly sprayed with non-stick cooking spray.
16. Arrange chicken breasts on top of dressing mixture.
17. Cover, bake at 350 degrees 45 minutes.
18. Remove cover, continue baking 5 to 10 minutes or until chicken breast registers internal temperature of 170 degrees.
19. Garnish with celery leaves, if desire.

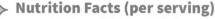

Nutrition Facts (per serving)
Calories 372 Carbohydrates 34 g
Protein 28 g Sodium 478 mg
Potassium 414 mg Phosphorus 204 mg

HEALTHY CHICKEN NUGGETS

Ingredients:
Based on 4 servings per recipe.
2 boneless, skinless chicken breasts, cubed
1/4 cup dijon mustard
1 cup panko bread crumbs
Directions:
1. Preheat oven to 500 degrees.
2. Pat chicken dry, cube into bite-size nugget pieces.
3. Dredge into mustard, then roll in bread crumbs.
4. Put on baking sheet, bake for 15 minutes.

Nutrition Facts (per serving)
Calories 247 Carbohydrates 20 g
Protein 31 g Sodium 484 mg
Potassium 384 mg Phosphorus 284 mg

SLOW COOKER GUMBO

Ingredients:
Based on 8 servings per recipe.
3 stalks celery, chopped
1 onion, chopped
3 boneless, skinless chicken breasts, chopped
2 cups low sodium chicken broth

4-8 ounces, sliced lean smoked turkey sausage
1/2 cup canola oil
1/2 cup flour
1 tablespoon Cajun Seasoning
1 red bell pepper, chopped
1/4 pounds cooked shrimp, optional
3 cups frozen, chopped okra, optional

Directions:
1. Add celery, onion, chicken and sausage to slow cooker.
2. Add low sodium chicken broth,
3. Add water if needed to cover chicken.
4. Let simmer 6-8 hours.
5. When you get home, put on the rice cooker, or start instant rice in a saucepan on the stove.
6. In frying pan, mix 1/2 cup canola oil and stir in 1/2 cup flour to make a roux.
7. Stir in Cajun seasoning and let cook for a minute or more depending on how dark you want your gumbo to be.
8. Slowly stir in some of the chicken broth from your slow cooker, stirring constantly to avoid lumps.
9. Once you have a thin paste, add it back to the slow cooker, along with cut-up red pepper, shrimp and okra (if you like it).
10. Cook for 10 minutes or until heated through and serve over rice.

Nutrition Facts (per serving)
Calories 306 Carbohydrates 14 g
Protein 20 g Sodium 503 mg
Potassium 335 mg Phosphorus 231 mg

SHRIMP SALAD WITH CUCUMBER MINT

Ingredients:
Based on 6 servings per recipe.
2 pounds medium shrimp, cleaned
1 cup fresh mint leaves
2 tablespoons lemon juice
3 tablespoons olive oil
1/2 English cucumber, seeded, diced
1 lemon lemon zest
pepper to taste

Directions:
1. Cook shrimp in boiling water for 3 minutes, drain and cool in refrigerator.
2. Put mint and lemon juice in food processor or blender and pulse to coarsely chop the mint.
3. Drizzle olive oil into processor while pureeing until mint is finely chopped.
4. In a serving bowl, toss shrimp, cucumber, mint mixture, zest, and pepper to combine.

Nutrition Facts (per serving)
Calories 229 Carbohydrates 3 g
Protein 31 g Sodium 226 mg
Potassium 357 mg Phosphorus 320 mg

MASTER MIX

Ingredients:
Based on 13 cups servings per recipe.
8 1/2 cups all-purpose flour
1 tablespoon baking powder
2 teaspoons cream of tartar
1 teaspoon baking soda
1 1/2 cups instant nonfat milk powder

2 1/4 cups vegetable shortening

Directions:

1. Sift together flour, baking powder, cream of tartar, baking soda, and milk powder.
2. Cut in shortening with a pastry blender until evenly distributed.
3. Store in a large, airtight container in a cool, dry place.
4. Use within 10-12 weeks.

About This Recipe

Use this low sodium and low phosphorus baking mix in any recipe that calls for Bisquick or other baking mix.

Nutrition Facts (per serving)

Calories 640 Carbohydrates 67 g
Protein 11 g Sodium 271 mg
Potassium 298 mg Phosphorus 189 mg

CHICKEN'N RICE

Ingredients:

Yield: 6 servings Serving size: ¾ cup
1 pound chicken parts
1 teaspoon black pepper
1 tablespoon poultry seasoning
½ cup chopped onion
1 teaspoon onion powder
½ teaspoon garlic powder
1 teaspoon crushed bay leaves (optional)
4 cups water
1 cup uncooked rice
1 tablespoon vegetable oil

Directions:

1. Place chicken parts, black pepper, poultry seasoning, onions, onion powder, garlic powder, and bay leaves in dutch

oven; cover with water. Cook until chicken is tender.
2. Remove chicken meat and skin from bone. Discard skin, reserve chicken meat and 2 cups of broth.
3. In a large pot, combine rice, vegetable oil, 2 cups broth, and chicken meat. Bring to a boil over medium-high heat.
4. Simmer on low heat for 20-25 minutes. Serve hot.

Nutrition Facts (per serving)

Calories 212 Carbohydrates 11 g
Protein 21 g Sodium 76 mg Fat 8 g
Potassium 283 mg Phosphorus 218 mg

TURKEY BURGERS

Ingredients:

Based on 4 servings per recipe.
1 pound lean ground turkey
1 cup (about 3 small) zucchini, grated
1 large egg
1/4 cup panko bread crumbs
1/4 cup red onion, grated
1 each garlic clove
1 teaspoon salt free seasoning
1/2 teaspoon black pepper
1 tablespoon vegetable oil

Directions:

1. In a large bowl, combine all ingredients. Mix well.
2. Form equal sized patties, about half inch thick.
3. In a large non-stick skillet, heat 1 teaspoon vegetable oil on medium high heat.

4. Add patties and reduce heat to low until browned, about 5 minutes each side.

5. Make sure patties are cooked through, no longer pink in the middle.

6. Freeze extras for a quick meal lat

Nutrition Facts (per serving)
Calories 176 Carbohydrates 8 g
Protein 31 g Sodium 98 mg Fat 3 g
Potassium 266 mg Phosphorus 62 mg

SEAFOOD CROQUETTES

Ingredients:
Yield: 8 patties Serving size: 1 patty
1 can water packed salmon or tuna (14.75-ounce), or 1 pound frozen or fresh crab meat.
2 egg whites
¼ cup chopped onion
½ teaspoon black pepper
½ cup plain bread crumb or unsalted cracker crumbs
1 tablespoon vegetable oil or cooking spray
2 tablespoons lemon juice (optional)
½ teaspoon ground mustard (crab only)
¼ cup regular mayonnaise (tuna and crab only)

Directions:
1. Drain water from canned meat.
2. Combine all ingredients except oil in a medium bowl. Mix well.
3. Form mixture into 8 separate balls, and then flatten to form patties.
4. Heat vegetable oil in skillet.
5. Place patties in hot oil.

6. Brown patties on each side. If cooked in oil, drain patties on paper towel.

Nutrition Facts (per serving)
Calories 189 Carbohydrates 11 g
Protein 14 g Sodium 337 mg Fat 8 g
Potassium 184 mg Phosphorus 191 mg

TUNA-NOOD LE SKILLET DINNER

Ingredients:
Yield: 4 servings Serving size: 1 cup vegetable cooking spray
2 tablespoons minced fresh onion
⅔ cup water
¼ teaspoon curry powder
¼ teaspoon black pepper
1 10 ¾-ounce can low sodium cream of mushroom soup, undiluted
2 cups hot cooked rotini (corkscrew pasta, cooked without salt or fat)
½ cup frozen green peas, thawed
1 9 ¼-ounce low sodium albacore tuna, with water, drained chopped fresh parsley (optional)

Directions:
1. Coat a large non-stick skillet with cooking spray; place over medium heat.
2. Add onion; sauté until tender.
3. Combine water, curry powder, pepper and soup in a bowl; stir well and add to skillet.
4. Add cooked rotini, peas, and tuna; stir well. Cook uncovered, over low heat 10 minutes, stirring occasionally.
5. Sprinkle with parsley, if desired.

Nutrition Facts (per serving)
Calories 269 Carbohydrates 38 g
Protein 18 g Sodium 407 mg
Potassium 515 mg Phosphorus 228 mg

SUPREME OF SEAFOOD

Ingredients:
Yield: 6 servings Serving size: ½ cup
1 cup crabmeat, cooked (boiled)
1 cup shrimp, cooked (boiled)
4 tablespoons green pepper, chopped
2 tablespoons green onions, chopped
1 cup celery, chopped
½ cup frozen green peas
½ teaspoon black pepper
½ cup mayonnaise
1 cup bread crumbs

Directions:
1. Preheat oven to 375ºF.
2. Combine all ingredients except bread crumbs in a bowl.
3. Place in a greased casserole dish.
4. Top with bread crumbs.
5. Bake for 30 minutes.

Nutrition Facts (per serving)
Calories 220 Carbohydrates 20 g
Protein 16 g Sodium 445 mg
Potassium 255 mg Phosphorus 148 mg

SPEEDY TORTILLA WRAPS

Ingredients:
Based on 6 servings per recipe.
4 ounces cream cheese

3 7" flour or corn tortillas
1 cup lettuce
4 ounces left over chicken, beef or fish
1 red bell pepper, sliced
1 tablespoon mayonnaise or low sodium ranch

Directions:
1. Spread cream cheese on tortilla.
2. Lay on lettuce leaves, meat, and pepper slices.
3. Spread with mayonnaise or low sodium ranch dressing.
4. Roll up each tortilla like a jelly roll.
5. Cut in half and wrap in plastic wrap to hold together.
6. Keep chilled in cooler for 6-8 hours.

Nutrition Facts (per serving)
Calories 184 Carbohydrates 14 g
Protein 9 g Sodium 233 mg
Potassium 156 mg Phosphorus 89 mg

RUSSIAN TEA

Ingredients:
Yield: 5 ½ cups dry powder/88 servings
Serving size: 1 tablespoon
2 cups Tang® ½ cup sugar
1 dry lemonade mix (2 quart size)
1 cup instant tea
1 teaspoon cloves
1 teaspoon cinnamon

Directions:
1. Combine all ingredients.
2. Store in a covered container.
3. To mix: add one tablespoon to 8-ounces hot water.
4. Serve hot.

Nutrition Facts (per serving)
Calories 54 Carbohydrates 13 g
Protein 0 g Sodium 0 mg
Potassium 25 mg Phosphorus 17 mg

GOBI CURRY

Ingredients:
Based on 4 servings per recipe.
2 tablespoons unsalted butter
1/2 medium yellow onion, finely chopped
1 teaspoon fresh ginger, minced
1/2 teaspoon turmeric
1/8 teaspoon cayenne pepper (optional)
1 teaspoon garam masala
2 cups cauliflower florets
1/2 cup frozen green peas
1 tablespoon water

Directions:
1. Heat butter in a medium saucepan over medium heat, add onions and cook until caramelized (soft and lightly browned).
2. Stir in ginger, turmeric, cayenne pepper and garam masala.
3. Stir in cauliflower and peas.
4. Add water and cover.
5. Reduce heat to low and steam for 10 minutes.

Nutrition Facts (per serving)
Calories 58 Carbohydrates 5 g
Protein 2 g Sodium 25 mg
Potassium 152 mg Phosphorus 27 mg

SWEDISH MEATBALLS

Ingredients:
Yield: 35 meatballs Serving size: 2 meatballs
Meatballs
1 pound lean
ground beef or turkey
¼ cup onions,
finely chopped
1 tablespoon lemon juice
1 teaspoon poultry seasoning (without salt)
1 teaspoon black pepper
¼ teaspoon dry mustard
¾ teaspoon onion powder
1 teaspoon italian seasoning
1 teaspoon granulated sugar
1 teaspoon Tabasco® sauce

Directions for meatballs:
1. Preheat oven to 425ºF.
2. Mix all ingredients together well.
3. Shape meatballs by using one tablespoon meat mixture for each meatball.
4. Place meatballs in a baking dish and bake for 20 minutes or until well done.
Make the sauce (recipe below).
5. Remove meatballs from oven and combine with sauce. Keep warm until ready to serve.
Sauce

Ingredients for sauce:
¼ cup vegetable oil
2 tablespoons all-purpose flour
1 teaspoon onion powder
2 teaspoons vinegar
2 teaspoons sugar
1 teaspoon Tabasco® sauce
2-3 cups water

Directions for sauce:
1. Combine oil and flour in saucepan; stir while cooking until golden brown. Remove from heat.
2. Add onion powder, vinegar, sugar, Tabasco® sauce, and water.
3. Return to heat, and continue stirring until thickened.

Nutrition Facts (per serving)
Calories 76 Carbohydrates 2 g
Protein 5 g Sodium 31 mg
Potassium 70 mg Phosphorus 44 mg

FIESTA LIME FAJITAS

Ingredients:
Yield: 5 servings Serving size: 2 drummettes
1 pound chicken drummettes
2 tablespoons olive oil
4 teaspoons Mrs.Dash® Fiesta Lime Seasoning Blend
1 pound chicken drummettes
2 tablespoons olive oil
4 teaspoons Mrs.Dash® Fiesta Lime Seasoning Blend
Directions:
1. Preheat oven to 350ºF.
2. Lightly brush the chicken drummettes with olive oil.
3. Sprinkle Mrs. Dash® Fiesta Lime Seasoning Blend on all sides.
4. Bake for 30 minutes or until chicken is cooked through.

Nutrition Facts (per serving)
Calories 100 Carbohydrates 0 g

Protein 18 g Sodium 35 mg
Potassium 105 mg Phosphorus 112 mg

STUFFED GREEN PEPPER

Ingredients:
Yield: 6 servings Serving size: 1 stuffed pepper
2 tablespoon vegetable oil
½ pound ground lean beef, turkey or chicken
¼ cup onions, chopped
¼ cup celery, chopped
2 tablespoons lemon juice
1 tablespoon celery seed
2 tablespoons italian seasoning
1 teaspoon black pepper
½ teaspoon sugar
1 ½ cups cooked rice
6 small green peppers, seeded with tops removed paprika
Directions:
1. Preheat oven to 325ºF.
2. Heat oil in saucepan.
3. Add ground meat, onions and celery, cook until meat is browned.
4. Add all ingredients except green peppers and paprika to sauce pan. Stir together, remove from heat.
5. Stuff peppers with mixture. Wrap with foil or place in a dish and cover. Bake for 30 minutes. Remove and sprinkle with paprika.

Nutrition Facts (per serving)
Calories 131 Carbohydrates 15 g
Protein 9 g Sodium 36 mg
Potassium 160 mg Phosphorus 83 mg

CONFETTI CHICKEN 'N RICE

Ingredients:

Based on 4 servings per recipe
3 tablespoons olive oil, divided
1 boneless, skinless chicken breast
3 ears, kernels removed or about 2 1/4 cups no salt added frozen corn
1 fresh zucchini, cubed
1 large red bell pepper, cubed
1 medium red onion, diced
1/2 teaspoon garlic powder
1 tablespoon cumin
1/2 teaspoon black pepper
2 teaspoons Mrs. Dash orginal
1/4 teaspoon cayenne pepper
1 package Uncle Ben's original ready rice

Directions:

1. In a large non-stick skillet heat 2 tablespoons olive oil on medium high heat.
2. When the oil is hot carefully place the chicken breast into the skillet.
3. When the juices run clear remove the chicken from the pan (about 15 minutes).
4. In the same skillet add 1 tablespoon olive oil and add corn, zucchini, red pepper, and onion.
5. Sautè on medium to medium high heat until the onions start to carmelize (about 10 minutes).
6. Next, add in garlic powder, cumin, black pepper, Mrs. dash, and cayenne pepper.
7. Cube chicken and return to the pan with the vegetables, reduce heat to medium low and keep stirring the mixture for about 5 minutes.
8. Follow the intructions on the rice package.
9. When the rice is done add it to the vegetables and continue to sautè for a few more minutes.
10. Serve and Enjoy!!

Nutrition Facts (per serving)
Calories 519 Carbohydrates 80 g
Protein 17 g Sodium 37 mg
Potassium 316 mg Phosphorus 152 mg

STIR FRY MEAL

Ingredients:

Yield: 3 servings Serving size: ½ cup chicken and vegetables with ⅔ cup rice
2 tablespoon cooking oil
2 medium chicken breast, cut in bite size pieces
1 10-ounce package frozen stir fry vegetables
½ tablespoon low sodium soy sauce
2 cups cooked rice

Directions:

1. Heat oil in 9-10" skillet on high.
2. Add chicken, and sauté.
3. Stir in vegetables.
4. Add soy sauce and stir well.
5. Reduce heat to medium high and cook uncovered for 3-5 minutes, or until done, stirring frequently.
6. Serve over ⅔ cup rice.

Calories 519 Carbohydrates 80 g
Protein 17 g Sodium 37 mg
Potassium 618 mg Phosphorus 26 mg

JALAPENO PEPPER CHICKEN

Ingredients:
Yield: 8 servings Serving size: 3-ounces
3 tablespoons vegetable oil
2-3 pounds chicken, cut up (skin and fat removed)
1 onion, sliced into rings
1 ½ cups low-sodium chicken bouillon
½ teaspoon ground nutmeg
¼ teaspoon black pepper
2 teaspoons fresh jalapeño peppers, finely chopped and seeded

Directions:
1. Heat oil, brown chicken pieces and set aside, keeping warm.
2. Add onion rings to oil and sauté. Add bouillon and bring to a boil, stirring often.
3. Return chicken to pan; add nutmeg and black pepper. Cover and simmer for 35 minutes or until chicken is tender.
4. Stir in jalapeño peppers, and simmer for another minute.

Nutrition Facts (per serving)
Calories 143 Carbohydrates 2 g
Protein 17 g Sodium 45 mg
Potassium 160 mg Phosphorus 127 mg

KICKIN' CHICKEN TACOS

Ingredients:
Based on 4 servings per recipe.
1 pound boneless, skinless chicken breasts
1 1/2 teaspoons salt-free taco seasoning
1 lime, juiced
8 corn tortillas
1 cup iceberg lettuce, shredded or chopped
1/4 cup sour cream
2 green onions (scallions), sliced
1/2 cup cilantro, chopped

Directions:
1. Boil chicken for 20 minutes.
2. Shred chicken into bite-size pieces or chop finely.
3. Toss chicken with Mexican seasoning and lime juice.
4. Fill tortillas with chicken and lettuce.
5. Top with sour cream, green onions, cilantro or other garnishes.

Nutrition Facts (per serving)
Calories 141 Carbohydrates 9 g
Protein 14 g Sodium 50 mg
Potassium 220 mg Phosphorus 155 mg

ORANGE-GLAZED CHICKEN

Ingredients:
Based on 6 servings per recipe.
1/4 cup oil
6 chicken breast halves
2 tablespoons flour
1/8 teaspoon nutmeg
1 dash ginger
1/4 teaspoon cinnamon
1 1/2 cup orange Juice
1/4 cup raisins
1/2 cup mandarin orange (optional)

Directions:
1. Heat oil in a non stick large fry pan.
2. Brown chicken on both sides.
3. Remove chicken and set aside.
4. Blend flour, nutmeg, ginger, and

cinnamon together; add mixture to hot oil.

5. Whisk together quickly to make a smooth paste.
6. Gradually add orange juice to pan.
7. Stir constantly.
8. Cook over medium heat until soft and thicken for 3 minutes.
9. Return chicken to pan.
10. Add raisins, cook on low heat for 30 minutes or until chicken is tender and fully cooked.
11. If sauce is too thick add water.
12. Add mandarin orange slice and heat until warm.

Nutrition Facts (per serving)
Calories 262 Carbohydrates 15 g
Protein 24 g Sodium 56 mg
Potassium 353 mg Phosphorus 182 mg

GRILLED PORK SOUVLAKI

Ingredients:
Yield: 8 servings Serving size: 1 skewer
1 bell green pepper
1 medium onion
2 garlic cloves
1 pound pork tenderloin or boneless pork loin chops
1/4 cup olive oil
3 tablespoons lemon juice
1 teaspoon dried whole oregano
1/8 teaspoon black pepper
Directions:
1. Cut bell peppper and onion into 2" cubes. Mince garlic cloves. Cut pork into 2" cubes.

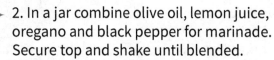

2. In a jar combine olive oil, lemon juice, oregano and black pepper for marinade. Secure top and shake until blended.
3. Place pork cubes in a bowl; pour marinade over and marinate in the refrigerator from 45 minutes up to 4 hours.
4. Thread bell pepper, pork and onion alternately on six 12" skewers.
5. Grill over medium-hot coals 12 to 15 minutes or to desired degree of doneness, turning half way though cooking.
Helpful hints
Protein requirements for those with kidney disease vary based on the stage of CKD. Check with your dietitian for adjustments to recipes or serving size based on your individual protein requirements.

Nutrition Facts (per serving)
Calories 204 Carbohydrates 5 g
Protein 18 g Sodium 58 mg
Potassium 336 mg Phosphorus 179 mg

DILLED FISH

Ingredients:
Based on 6 servings per recipe.
1 1/2 pounds fresh, firm white fish
1 teaspoon instant (freeze dried) onion, minced
1/4 teaspoon mustard powder
1/2 teaspoon dill weed
a dash of pepper
4 teaspoons lemon juice

Directions:
1. Preheat oven to 475 degrees.
2. Rinse fish and pat it dry.
3. Arrange in baking dish.
4. Combine onion, mustard, dill weed, and pepper in 2 tablespoons water.
5. Add lemon juice to spice and pour evenly over fish.
6. Bake uncovered for 17-20 minutes.

Nutrition Facts (per serving)
Calories 112 Carbohydrates 1 g
Protein 23 g Sodium 63 mg
Potassium 350 mg Phosphorus 194 mg

CRAB CAKES

Ingredients:
Yield: 6 servings Serving size: 1 patty
1 egg (egg substitute or egg white optional)
⅓ cup green or red pepper, finely chopped
⅓ cup low sodium crackers
¼ cup reduced fat mayonnaise
1 tablespoon dry mustard
1 teaspoon crushed red pepper or black pepper
2 tablespoons lemon juice
1 teaspoon garlic powder
2 tablespoon vegetable oil
Directions:
1. Combine all ingredients.
2. Divide into 6 balls and form patties.
3. Heat vegetable oil in pan at medium heat or oven at 350ºF.
4. Fry patties 4-5 minutes or bake 15 minutes in oven.
5. Serve warm.

Nutrition Facts (per serving)
Calories 101 Carbohydrates 5 g
Protein 2 g Sodium 67 mg
Potassium 72 mg Phosphorus 43 mg

FIESTA LIME TACOS

Ingredients:
Yield: 12 servings Serving size: 1 taco
1 pound of lean ground beef or turkey
4 tablespoons Mrs. Dash® Fiesta Lime Seasoning Blend
¾ cup water 12 taco shells or 6" flour tortillas
Directions:
1. Brown ground meat in a large skillet on medium-high heat.
2. Drain excess fat. 3. Stir in Mrs. Dash® Fiesta Lime Seasoning Blend and water.
4. Bring to a boil. Reduce heat and simmer 5 minutes, stirring occasionally.
5. Spoon into warm taco shells or tortillas. Serve with toppings, if desired.

Nutrition Facts (per serving)
Calories 140 Carbohydrates 9 g
Protein 7 g Sodium 70 mg
Potassium 140 mg Phosphorus 111 mg

BASIC MEAT LOAF

Ingredients:
Yield: 8 servings Serving size: 2-ounces
1 pound lean ground turkey
1 egg white
1 tablespoon lemon juice
½ cup plain bread crumbs

½ teaspoon onion powder
½ teaspoon italian seasoning
¼ teaspoon black pepper
½ cup chopped onions
½ cup diced green bell pepper
¼ cup water

Directions:
1. Preheat oven to 400ºF.
2. Pour lemon juice over meat.
3. In a bowl combine remaining ingredients.
4. Add to meat and mix well.
5. Place in a loaf pan; bake for 45 minutes.

Nutrition Facts (per serving)
Calories 110 Carbohydrates 2 g
Protein 12 g Sodium 71 mg
Potassium 138 mg Phosphorus 87 mg

CIDER CREAM CHICKEN

Ingredients:
Based on 8 servings per recipe.
4 bone-in chicken breasts
2 tablespoons unsalted butter
3/4 cup apple cider
1/2 cup half and half

Directions:
1. Melt butter over medium-high heat. Add chicken and brown on both sides.
2. Add cider and reduce heat to medium; simmer for about 20 minutes.
3. Remove chicken from skillet.
4. Boil cider until reduced to about 1/4 cup.
5. Add half and half over heat; whisk until slightly thickened.
6. Pour cream sauce over chicken and serve.

Nutrition Facts (per serving)
Calories 186 Carbohydrates 1 g
Protein 27 g Sodium 83 mg
Potassium 414 mg Phosphorus 266 mg

BAKED FISH

Ingredients:
Yield: 4 servings Serving size: 3-ounces
4 3-ounce trout fillets or any other baking fish
1 ½ teaspoon black pepper
1 tablespoon garlic powder
1 ½ teaspoon paprika
¼ medium green pepper
1 small onion
1 small lemon
2 tablespoons parmesan cheese

Directions:
1. Preheat oven to 375ºF.
2. Place fish in a greased baking pan or on aluminum foil.
3. Sprinkle black pepper, garlic powder, and paprika on both sides of fish.
4. Cut green peppers into strips and place on fish. Slice onions into rings and place on fish.
5. Squeeze juice of lemon onto fish.
6. Bake for 30 minutes.
7. After fish has cooked, sprinkle with parmesan cheese. Serve hot.

Nutrition Facts (per serving)
Calories 164 Carbohydrates 8 g
Protein 20 g Sodium 86 mg
Potassium 452 mg Phosphorus 252 mg

CURRY CHICKEN

Ingredients:
Yield: 6 servings Serving size:
3-ounces
1 whole chicken, skin removed, cut in small parts.
¼ cup lemon juice
2 teaspoons curry powder
1 medium onion, chopped
1 medium garlic glove, chopped (optional)
½ teaspoon black pepper
½ teaspoon dry thyme
2 tablespoon vegetable or olive oil 1 cup water

Directions:
1. Wash cleaned chicken in lemon juice.
2. Mix seasoning together and rub on to chicken parts.
3. Allow to marinate in refrigerator for 1 hour (preferable overnight).
4. Heat oil in a saucepan, sauté seasoned chicken until browned.
5. Rinse remainder seasoning from marinated pan with water.
6. Pour over browned chicken. Let simmer until tender.
7. Serve over hot rice.

Nutrition Facts (per serving)
Calories 323 Carbohydrates 5 g
Protein 21 g Sodium 93 mg
Potassium 317 mg Phosphorus 214 mg

CHICKEN STEW

Ingredients:
Yield: 6 servings Serving size: 1 cup
3 tablespoon vegetable oil
2 pounds chicken breast cut in bite size pieces
1 cup sliced onions
¾ cup green peppers
2 cloves garlic, minced
2 tablespoon all-purpose flour
2 10 ½-ounce cans low-sodium chicken broth
1 10-ounce bag frozen carrots
¼ teaspoon dried basil
¼ teaspoon black pepper
1 110-ounce bag frozen sliced okra cup water

Directions:
1. Heat 2 tablespoons of oil in dutch oven; add chicken and sauté over medium high heat.
2. Remove chicken and set aside. Add remaining 1 tablespoon of oil
3. Add and sauté onion, pepper and garlic.
4. Add flour and cook 2-3 minutes, stirring constantly.
5. Add chicken and broth, cook until boiling.
6. Add carrots, basil and black pepper, cover and simmer for about 10 minutes. Gravy will thicken as it simmers.
7. Add okra and cook for 5-10 more minutes.
8. Serve over hot white rice.

Nutrition Facts (per serving)
Calories 142 Carbohydrates 13 g
Protein 10 g Sodium 93 mg

Potassium 453 mg Phosphorus 129 mg

PARSLEY BURGER

Ingredients:
Yield: 4 servings Serving size: 1 patty,
3-ounces
1 pound lean ground beef or ground
turkey
1 tablespoon lemon juice
1 tablespoon parsley flakes
¼ teaspoon black pepper
¼ teaspoon ground thyme
¼ teaspoon oregano

Directions:
1. Mix all ingredients thoroughly.
2. Shape into 4 small patties about ¾"
thick.
3. Place on lightly greased skillet
or broiler pan.
4. Broil about 3" from the heat for 10-15
minutes, turning once.

Nutrition Facts (per serving)
Calories 171 Carbohydrates 0 g
Protein 20 g Sodium 108 mg
Potassium 289 mg Phosphorus 180 mg

OVEN FRIED CHICKEN

Ingredients:
Yield: 8 servings (or 8 pieces) Serving size:
3 or 4-ounces
2 ½ pound fryer (cut as desired)
1 tablespoon lemon juice
1 cup all-purpose flour

1 teaspoon black pepper
1 cup corn flakes, crushed
¼ teaspoon poultry seasoning
4 tablespoons vegetable oil

Directions:
1. Preheat oven to 400ºF.
2. Wash chicken parts thoroughly and pat
dry; rub with lemon juice.
3. In a small bag, combine flour, black
pepper, corn flakes, and poultry
seasoning. Shake well.
4. In a shallow baking pan (about 1"
deep), grease with vegetable oil.
5. Place chicken in bag of ingredients,
using the largest pieces first. Shake well.
6. Arrange coated chicken in pan.
7. Brown in oven 20-30 minutes on each
side.

Nutrition Facts (per serving)
Calories 280 Carbohydrates 15 g
Protein 15 g Sodium 74 mg
Potassium 150 mg Phosphorus 120 mg

NEW ORLEANS-STYLE RICE DRESSING

Ingredients:
Yield: 4 servings Serving size: 1 cup
2 tablespoons vegetable oil
¼ cup green peppers, chopped
1 pound lean ground turkey
½ teaspoon cayenne pepper
2 tablespoons all-purpose flour
1 clove garlic, chopped
¼ cup onion, chopped 2 cups hot
cooked rice
¼ cup green onions, chopped
1 cup low sodium chicken broth

¼ cup celery, chopped
Directions:
1. Heat oven to 350 ºF.
2. Heat oil in skillet, add meat and cook on medium heat until browned.
3. Remove meat and drain on paper towel.
4. Add flour to skillet and brown to make a dark roux.
5. Add onions, celery, peppers and garlic to roux and cook until vegetables are tender.
6. Add cooked rice and meat to skillet.
7. Add low sodium broth a little at a time until mixture is moist. If mixture is too dry may add water.
8. Pour into a 1 ½ quart baking dish.
9. Bake for 20 minutes

Nutrition Facts (per serving)
Calories 393 Carbohydrates 28 g
Protein 27 g Sodium 113 mg
Potassium 377 mg Phosphorus 228 mg

FAJITAS

Ingredients:
Yield: 4 servings Serving size: 4 medium strips
2 tablespoon vegetable oil 1 ½ pounds raw chicken strips or beef strips or shrimp peeled and deveined)
2 teaspoon chili powder
½ teaspoon cumin
2 tablespoon lemon or lime juice
¼ green and/or red pepper, sliced lengthwise
½ onion white, sliced lengthwise
½ teaspoon dry cilantro

4 flour tortillas vegetable spray
Directions:
1. Preheat oven to 300ºF.
2. Add vegetable oil to non-stick frying pan over medium heat.
3. Add meat, seasonings and lemon/lime juice; cook for 5-10 minutes or until tender.
4. Add pepper and onion to pan and cook 1-2 minutes.
5. Remove from heat; add cilantro.
6. Place tortillas on foil and move to oven. Heat for 10 minutes
7. Divide mixture
between tortillas, wrap and serve.

Nutrition Facts (per serving)
Calories 184 Carbohydrates 5 g
Protein 19 g Sodium 121 mg
Potassium 494 mg Phosphorus 207 mg

TACO STUFFING

Ingredients:
Yield: 8 servings Serving size: 2-ounces stuffing in each shell
2 tablespoon vegetable oil
1 ¼ pounds lean ground beef or turkey
½ teaspoon ground red pepper
½ teaspoon black pepper
1 teaspoon italian seasoning
1 teaspoon garlic powder
1 teaspoons onion powder
½ teaspoon Tabasco® sauce
½ teaspoon nutmeg Will also need: 1 medium taco shells
½ head shredded lettuce
Directions:
1. Heat oil. Place ground meat and all

remaining ingredients except taco shells and lettuce in a skillet. Cook until beef is done and ingredients are well-blended.
2. Stuff taco shells with 2-ounces of meat and top with shredded lettuce.

Nutrition Facts (per serving)
Calories 176 Carbohydrates 9 g
Protein 14 g Sodium 124 mg
Potassium 258 mg Phosphorus 150 mg

SALISBURY STEAK

Ingredients:
Yield: 4 servings Serving size: 3-ounce
1 pound chopped steak or lean ground beef, chicken or turkey
1 small onion, chopped
½ cup green pepper, chopped
1 teaspoon black pepper
1 egg
1 tablespoon vegetable oil
½ cup water
1 tablespoon corn starch
Directions:
1. Mix together meat, onion, green pepper, black pepper, and egg. Form into patties.
2. Heat oil in skillet, add patties and cook on both sides.
3. Add half of water and simmer for 15 minutes. Remove patties.
4. To meat drippings, add remaining water and corn starch. Simmer while stirring to thicken gravy.
5. Pour gravy over steak and serve hot.

Nutrition Facts (per serving)
Calories 249 Carbohydrates 7 g
Protein 22 g Sodium 128 mg
Potassium 366 mg Phosphorus 218 mg

FISH TACOS

Ingredients:
Yield: 4 servings Serving size: 3 ½-ounce
12-16 fish fillets (1 pound), tilapia or as desired
20 saltine crackers, unsalted tops, crushed finely
¼ cup unsalted butter or margarine
2 teaspoon dill weed
1 teaspoon garlic powder
¼ cup lemon juice
Directions:
1. Preheat oven to 400ºF.
2. Combine crackers, garlic and dill.
3. Melt butter or margarine.
4. Roll fish in melted butter, then in crumbs and again in butter mix.
5. Place in baking pan and bake 8-10 minutes untill fish is flakey.

Nutrition Facts (per serving)
Calories 164 Carbohydrates 7 g
Protein 21 g Sodium 138 mg
Potassium 335 mg Phosphorus 181 mg

FAST FAJITAS

Ingredients:
Based on 4 (2 fajitas each) servings per recipe.
1 tablespoon olive oil
1 lime juice and zest of lime
1 lemon juice and zest of lemon or orange
1 teaspoon cumin
dash cayenne pepper
1 pound meat, shrimp, tofu, bite size pieces
1 onion, sliced
2 bell peppers, sliced
8 corn tortillas
sour cream to taste
cilantro to taste

Directions:
1. Combine oil, citrus zest and juice, cumin, and cayenne pepper in a small bowl to make the marinade.
2. Place meat, vegetables, and marinade in a bag or shallow dish and marinate overnight.
3. In a large skillet over medium heat, cook marinated meat and vegetables until the onions become soft and begin to caramalize (turn light brown) and the meat is cooked through. This should take at least 15-20 minutes.
4. Serve in tortillas and top with sour cream and cilantro

Nutrition Facts (per serving)
Calories 320 Carbohydrates 34 g
Protein 29 g Sodium 142 mg
Potassium 445 mg Phosphorus 332 mg

SPICY LAMB

Ingredients:
Yield: 4 servings Serving size: 3-ounces
¼ cup vegetable oil
1 ½ tablespoons garlic powder
3 teaspoons dry mustard
1 leg of lamb (trimmed for roasting)

Directions:
1. Blend ingredients for marinade: oil, garlic powder and mustard.
2. Coat leg of lamb with marinade; refrigerate 6-8 hours or overnight.
3. Adjust meat on barbecue spit and roast for 30 minutes per pound or until 170°F on meat thermometer, basting meat continuously with marinade.

Nutrition Facts (per serving)
Calories 289 Carbohydrates 3 g
Protein 24 g Sodium 144 mg
Potassium 423 mg Phosphorus 237 mg

ONE-POT CHICKEN AND DUMPLINGS

Ingredients:
Yield: 6 servings Serving size: 1 cup
5 Tablespoons cold unsalted butter, divided
1 small yellow onion, minced
1 stalk celery, thinly sliced
2 carrots, diced medium
1 1/4 cup all-purpose flour, divided
3 cups low sodium chicken broth (*see note)
1–2 cups diced cooked chicken
1/3 pound green beans, trimmed and cut into 1-inch pieces (or just use frozen

green beans)
Opt spices (we think these make the recipe go from good to wow!)
1 bay leaf
1 tablespoon parsley
1/4 tsp celery seed
1/2 tsp rosemary
1/2 tsp thyme
3 drop sriracha sauce
Pepper to taste
1 teaspoon baking powder
2 tablespoons chopped fresh parsley, plus more for topping
1/2 cup unsweetened almond milk or rice milk

Directions:

1. In a large saucepan, melt 3 tablespoons butter over medium-high. Add onion, celery, and carrots and cook until onion is translucent, about 4 minutes. Add 1/4 cup flour and cook, stirring, 1 minute. Gradually add broth, stirring constantly, then bring to a boil. Reduce heat and simmer 5 minutes. Stir in chicken, green beans, spices and season with salt and pepper.
2. Make dumplings: Whisk together 1 cup flour, baking powder, 1/2 tsp coarse salt (opt), and 2 tablespoons parsley. Cut in 2 tablespoons butter. Stir in almond milk. Drop heaping spoonfuls batter on top of chicken mixture. Cover and simmer until dumplings are cooked through, about 12 minutes. Serve topped with additional chopped parsley.

Notes

*Look carefully at your label for your broth and stock. They vary widely in potassium and sodium content. * I added a 1/2 tsp salt after tasting it. This adds

~200 mg sodium/serving. You may not need this, and ideally you'd leave it out. However, in perspective 366 mg sodium for a cup of soup is very reasonable for a meal.

Nutrition Facts (per serving)
Calories 230 Carbohydrates 30 g
Protein 5 g Sodium 146 mg
Potassium 455 mg Phosphorus 227 mg

CRUNCHY CHICKEN NUGGETS

Ingredients:
Yield: 8 servings Serving size: 2-ounces
2 egg whites
1 tablespoon water
2 ½ cups ready-to-eat crispy rice cereal
1 ½ teaspoons paprika
¼ teaspoon seasoning salt
⅛ teaspoon garlic powder
⅛ teaspoon onion powder
1 pound boneless, skinless chicken breasts
1 tablespoon butter or margarine, melted
1 tablespoon reduced-fat ranch dressing (for dipping)

Directions:
1. In a shallow dish combine egg whites and water.
2. On a large sheet of wax paper combine crispy rice cereal, paprika, seasoning salt, garlic powder and onion powder.
3. Cut chicken into 1 ½" pieces.
4. Dip chicken into egg white mixture, coating all sides. Roll in cerealmixture.
5. Place in a single layer on ungreased baking sheet. Drizzle with melted butter.

6. Bake at 450ºF for about 12 minutes or until no longer pink in center.
7. Serve warm with dipping sauce (reduced-fat ranch dressing).

Nutrition Facts (per serving)
Calories 122 Carbohydrates 8 g
Protein 14 g Sodium 176 mg
Potassium 237 mg Phosphorus 134 mg

ROSEMARY, LEMON, AND MUSTARD MARINADE

Ingredients:
Based on 6 servings per recipe.
1/2 cup lemon juice
3 tablespoons dijon mustard
2 tablespoons honey
1 tablespoon fresh rosemary, minced
Directions:
1. In large bowl or big zip lock bag, mix together lemon juice, mustard, honey, and minced rosemary.
2. Add poultry or fish and turn to evenly coat.
3. Cover or close tightly, and chill at least 30 minutes or up to a day; stir or turn occasionally.
4. Drain poultry or fish and discard the marinade.
5. Grill poultry or fish over indirect heat.
6. Garnish with fresh rosemary sprigs

Nutrition Facts (per serving)
Calories 35 Carbohydrates 9 g
Protein 1 g Sodium 180 mg
Potassium 46 mg Phosphorus 2 mg

TURKEY & NOODLES

Ingredients:
Yield: 8 servings Serving size: 1 cup.
2 cups dry elbow macaroni
1 tablespoon vegetable or olive oil
2 pounds fresh lean ground turkey
½ cup green onions, chopped
½ cup green pepper, chopped
1 14-ounce can regular diced tomatoes
1 tablespoon italian seasoning
1 teaspoon black pepper
Directions:
1. Cook macaroni in medium boiler in 4 cups of boiling water. Allow to boil for 5 minutes or desired tenderness. Drain and set a side.
2. Heat vegetable oil in a large skillet over medium heat. Add ground turkey and cook until done, stirring occasionally.
3. Add onions, green peppers, diced tomatoes, italian seasoning, black pepper and cooked macaroni. Mix well.
4. Cover and let simmer for 5 minutes or until desired. Serve warm.

Nutrition Facts (per serving)
Calories 273 Carbohydrates 22 g
Protein 33 g Sodium 188 mg
Potassium 533 mg Phosphorus 296 mg

STRIP STEAK WITH SMOTHERED ONIONS

Ingredients:
Yield: 6 servings Serving size: 2 oz steak, about 1/3 cup onions
1/4 tsp black pepper
1 tbsp olive oil(divided)

2 sweet onion(peeled and halved, thinly sliced)
1/4 cup water
1/2 tsp salt
1/2 tsp dried thyme
1/2 tsp brown sugar
1 lb lean strip steak

Directions:

1. Sprinkle the steak with the salt and pepper.
2. Heat 1/2 Tbsp of the oil in a large cast-iron skillet over high heat. Add the steak and sear for about 3 minutes. Turn the steak over, reduce the heat to medium, and cook for 4 to 6 minutes, or longer as desired for doneness. Remove the steak from the pan and keep it warm.
3. Add the remaining oil to the pan. Add the onions and sauté over medium heat for 5 minutes. Add the water, thyme, and brown sugar, cover the pan, and simmer over medium-low heat for 10 minutes, until the onions are very soft.
4. Slice the steak. Serve the slices covered with the onions.

Nutrition Facts (per serving)
Calories 170 Carbohydrates 9 g
Protein 18 g Sodium 200 mg
Potassium 360 mg Phosphorus 200 mg

BEEF OR CHICKEN ENCHILADAS

Ingredients:
Based on 6 servings per recipe.
1 pound lean ground beef or chicken
1/2 cup onion, chopped

1 teaspoon cumin
1/2 teaspoon black pepper
1 garlic clove, chopped
12 corn tortillas
1 can enchilada sauce

Directions:

1. Preheat oven to 375 degrees.
2. Brown meat in frying pan.
3. Add onion, garlic, cumin and pepper. Continue cooking. Stir until onions are soft.
4. In another pan fry tortillas in a small amount of oil.
5. Dip each tortilla in enchilada sauce.
6. Fill with meat mixture and roll up.
7. Place enchilada in a shallow pan and top with sauce and cheese if desired.
8. Bake until cheese is melted and enchiladas are golden brown.

Nutrition Facts (per serving)
Calories 235 Carbohydrates 30 g
Protein 13 g Sodium 201 mg
Potassium 222 mg Phosphorus 146 mg

PASTA WITHOUT TOMATO SAUCE

Ingredients:
Yield: 2 servings Serving size: 2
2 Tbsp extra-virgin olive oil
6 cloves Garlic (thinly sliced)
1/2 small Red Onion (minced)
1/4 cup Dried Cranberries
4 cups Kale, fresh (torn or thinly sliced)
1/4 cup Water
4 oz, dry Spaghetti Noodles (Choose white or wheat noodles. Potassium

and phosphorus content differs in these two products.)

1/4 cup, sliced and pitted Kalamata Olives

2 Tbsp, crumbled Feta Cheese

Directions:

1. Heat olive oil over medium-high heat in a large skillet. Add garlic slices then cook, stirring near constantly, until slices are pale golden brown. Remove to a plate and set aside.

2. Turn heat down to medium then add red onion. Season with salt and pepper then cook until golden-brown and tender, about 3 minutes. Add cranberries and kale, season with more salt and pepper, then add water, place a lid on top of the skillet and cook for 4-5 minutes, or until kale is tender.

3. Add spaghetti to a large pot of salted, boiling water then cook until al dente.

4. Add kalamata olives to cooked kale and cranberry mixture. Transfer cooked spaghetti to skillet then toss to combine all ingredients. Add up to 1/4 cup pasta cooking water if needed. Divide between two plates then top with 1 Tablespoon feta cheese and half the cooked garlic slices each.

Nutrition Facts (per serving)
Calories 271 Carbohydrates 27,5 g
Protein 4 g Sodium 227 mg
Potassium 269 mg Phosphorus 89 mg

MEDITERRANEAN LAMB PATTIES

Ingredients:
Based on 4 servings per recipe.
1 lb. ground lamb
1 whole egg
1/4 cup panko* bread crumbs
1/4 cup onion, finely chopped
1 clove garlic, finely chopped
1 teaspoon dried oregano (or dried mint)
1/2 teaspoon ground pepper
1/2 cup feta cheese, crumbled

Directions:

1. In a large bowl, combine all ingredients, mixing well.

2. Form into four equal sized patties, about 1/2 inch thick.

3. Preheat a large non-stick skillet over medium-high heat.

4. Add patties and keep the heat high until browned, then flip, about 5 minutes each side and turn down the heat.

5. Be sure patties are cooked all the way through, no longer pink in the middle or when internal temperature reaches 160 degrees.

Nutrition Facts (per serving)
Calories 305 Carbohydrates 5 g
Protein 19 g Sodium 229 mg
Potassium 45 mg Phosphorus 74 mg

FISH STICKS

Ingredients:
Yield: 8 servings Serving size: 2 strips
cooking spray

1 cup whole wheat, plain, or Panko dry breadcrumbs
1 cup whole grain or plain cereal flakes
1 teaspoon lemon pepper
½ teaspoon garlic powder
½ teaspoon paprika
¼ teaspoon salt
2 large egg whites, beaten
½ cup all-purpose flour
3 tilapia fillets (1 pound), cut into ½ by 3" strips

Directions:
1. Preheat oven to 450ºF.
2. Set a wire rack on a baking sheet; coat with cooking spray.
3. Place breadcrumbs, cereal flakes, lemon pepper, garlic powder, paprika, and salt in a food processor or blender. Process until finely ground. Transfer to a shallow dish.
4. Place beaten egg whites in a second shallow dish and flour in a third shallow dish.
5. Dredge each strip of fish in the flour, dip it in the egg and then coat all sideswith the breadcrumb mixture. Place on the prepared rack. Coat both sides of the breaded fish with cooking spray.
6. Bake until golden brown and crisp, about 10 minutes.

Tip: Panko breadcrumbs are known for their coarse and crunchy texture onù baked foods.

Nutrition Facts (per serving)
Calories 154 Carbohydrates 19 g
Protein 15 g Sodium 240 mg
Potassium 224 mg Phosphorus 130 mg

OPEN-FACED STEAK & ONION SANDWICH

Ingredients:
Yield: 4 servings Serving size: 3-ounces
4 chopped steaks (4-ounces each)
1 tablespoon lemon juice
1 tablespoon italian seasoning
1 tablespoon black pepper
1 tablespoon vegetable oil
1 medium onion, sliced into rings
4 hoagie rolls, sliced

Directions:
1. Combine meat with lemon juice, italian seasoning and black pepper.
2. Heat oil in frying pan over medium heat.
3. Brown seasoned steaks on both sides until tender. Remove and drain on paper towels.
4. Lower heat; add onion and sauté until onions are tender.
5. Serve open-faced on sliced hoagie roll, topped with onion rings.

Nutrition Facts (per serving)
Calories 345 Carbohydrates 26 g
Protein 14 g Sodium 247 mg
Potassium 200 mg Phosphorus 115 mg

ROTINI WITH MOCK ITALIAN SAUSAGE

Ingredients:
Yield: 4 servings Serving size: ¾ cups turkey mixture and 1 cup rotini
4 ounces uncooked rotini pasta
¾ pound lean ground turkey

1 cup onion, chopped
1 clove garlic, minced
½ cup chopped celery
¾ teaspoon italian seasoning
¼ teaspoon fennel seeds
¼ teaspoon crushed red pepper
3 tablespoons tomato paste
1-14 ½ unsalted can (190 grams) tomatoes, chopped
2 tablespoons grated parmesan cheese

Directions:
1. Boil rotini pasta according to package directions, drain.
2. Sauté turkey in a non-stick skillet over medium heat until browned,stirring to crumble. Drain on paper towel.
3. Add onion, garlic, celery, and seasonings. Cook 3 minutes; stirring occasionally.
4. Add tomato paste and tomatoes. Partially cover, reduce heat, and simmer 15 minutes.
5. Serve over rotini. Top with cheese.

Nutrition Facts (per serving)
Calories 165 Carbohydrates 28 g
Protein 13 g Sodium 250 mg
Potassium 458 mg Phosphorus 161 mg

DIJON CHICKEN

Ingredients:
Based on 4 servings per recipe.
4 boneless chicken breasts
1/4 cup Dijon mustard
3 tablespoons honey
1 teaspoon lemon Juice
1 teaspoon curry powder
Directions:

1. Preheat oven to 350 degrees.
2. Place chicken in a baking dish.
3. In a bowl mix together other ingredients.
4. Brush both side of chicken with sauce.
5. Bake for 30 minutes or until chicken reaches an internal temperature of 165 degrees.

Nutrition Facts (per serving)
Calories 189 Carbohydrates 14 g
Protein 25 g Sodium 258 mg
Potassium 454 mg Phosphorus 250 mg

EGGPLANT CASSEROLE

Ingredients:
Yield: 8 servings Serving size: ½ cup
1 large eggplant
2 tablespoon vegetable oil
½ cup green pepper, chopped
½ cup onion, finely chopped
1 pound lean ground beef or turkey
2 cups plain bread crumbs
1 large egg, slightly beaten
½ teaspoon red pepper, optional
Directions:
1. Preheat oven to 350ºF.
2. Boil eggplant until tender; drain and mash.
3. Heat oil; add green pepper, onion and ground meat. Sauté until cooked.
4. Add eggplant, bread crumbs and egg, mixing well.
5. Add red pepper to taste, if desired.
6. Bake in casserole dish for 30-45 ù minutes. Serve warm.

CHICKEN SEAFOOD GUMBO

Ingredients:
Based on 12, one cup servings per recipe.
1 tablespoon canola oil
3 celery stalks, chopped
1 yellow onion, chopped
1 red bell pepper, chopped
2 skinless chicken breasts, chopped
8 ounces lean smoked turkey sausage, sliced
1/2 cup canola oil
1/2 cup flour
1 tablespoon salt-free Cajun seasoning
2 quarts low sodium chicken broth
1/2 pound cooked shrimp
6 ounces canned crab, drained
3 cups frozen okra, chopped

Directions:
1. Heat 1 tablespoon canola oil in a 4.5 quart or larger pot over medium heat.
2. Add celery, onion, bell pepper, chicken, and sausage and cook for 10 minutes.
3. Remove mixture from pot and set aside.
4. Reduce heat to medium.
5. Add 1/2 cup canola oil and stir in flour to make a roux.
6. Stir in Cajun seasoning and let cook for a minute or more depending on how dark you want your gumbo to be.
7. Very slowly stir in chicken broth, stirring constantly to avoid lumps.
8. Increase heat to medium-high and bring mixture to a boil and let boil for about 10 minutes or until it starts to thicken slightly.
9. Reduce heat to medium and add shrimp, crab, and okra, and add chicken mixture back into pot as well.
10. Cook for 10 minutes or until heated through.

PASTA WITH PESTO

Ingredients:
Yield: 6 servings Serving size 1 cup
16 oz White Pasta
2 medium Zucchini, sliced into half moons
1 medium Yellow Squash, sliced into half moons
1 Large Red Bell Pepper, diced inch squares
1/2 cup Mushrooms, sliced fairly thick
2 tbsp Olive Oil
2 cloves Garlic
2/3 cup Pesto Sauce
1/4 cup Feta Cheese

Directions:
1. Preheat oven to 425 degrees.
2. Place zucchini, squash, bell pepper, onion and mushrooms on 18 by 13 inch baking sheet.
3. Drizzle veggies with olive oil then toss to evenly coat.

4. Roast in preheated oven until veggies tender.
5. While veggies are roasting cook pasta according to package and drain.
6. Pour drained pasta into a large bowl.
7. Add in roasted veggies and pesto then toss to evenly coat.
8. Serve warm.

Nutrition Facts (per serving)
Calories 492 Carbohydrates 67 g
Protein 13,4 g Sodium 336 mg
Potassium 476 mg Phosphorus 237 mg

BARBECUE CUPS

Ingredients:
Yield: 10 servings Serving size: 1 biscuit
¾ pounds lean ground turkey
½ cup spicy barbecue sauce
2 teaspoons onion flakes dash garlic powder
1 10-ounces package low-fat refrigerator biscuits
Directions:
1. Brown turkey.
2. Add barbecue
sauce, onion flakes and garlic powder. Mix well.
3. Flatten each biscuit and press into muffin tin.
4. Spoon beef mixture into center of each biscuit cup.
5. Bake at 400ºF for 10 to 12 minutes.

Nutrition Facts (per serving)
Calories 134 Carbohydrates 13 g
Protein 7 g Sodium 342 mg

Potassium 151 mg Phosphorus 152 mg

CREAMY TUNA TWIST

Ingredients:
Based on 4-1 cup servings per recipe.
3/4 cup mayonnaise
2 tablespoons vinegar
1 1/2 cups shell macaroni, cooked
1 can (6 1/2 ounces) tuna *unsalted or water packed, drained
1/2 cup peas, cooked
1/2 cup celery, chopped pea size
1 tablespoon dried dill weed
Directions:
1. Stir mayonnaise, vinegar, and macaroni shells together in a large bowl until smooth.
2. Add remaining ingredients, stir until combined.
3. Cover and chill.

Nutrition Facts (per serving)
Calories 421 Carbohydrates 20 g
Protein 15 g Sodium 379 mg
Potassium 204 mg Phosphorus 122 mg

BROCCOLI CHICKEN CASSEROLE

Ingredients:
Based on 6 servings per recipe.
2-3 cups cooked broccoli
1 medium onion, chopped
2-3 chicken breast, diced
2 tablespoons butter or margarine

2 eggs, beaten
2 cups milk
2 cups cooked rice, barley, or noodles
2 cups grated cheese
grated parmesan to top

Directions:

1. Preheat oven to 350 degrees.
2. Place broccoli in microwavable bowl, cover with plastic wrap and microwave until bright green, about 2-3 minutes.
3. Meanwhile, brown onion and chicken in butter in a pan.
4. Mix all ingredients and put in greased casserole dish.
5. Sprinkle top with grated parmesan and bake about 1 hour and 15 minutes, until set and fork comes out clean.

Nutrition Facts (per serving)
Calories 368 Carbohydrates 26 g
Protein 26 g Sodium 388 mg
Potassium 371 mg Phosphorus 243 mg

ALASKA BAKED MACARONI AND CHEESE

Ingredients:
Based on 8 servings per recipe.
3 cups elbow, small shell or bowtie pasta
2 tablespoons flour
2 tablespoons unsalted butter
2 cups milk
1 teaspoon mustard powder
1 teaspoon paprika
1 tablespoon fresh thyme or tarragon, chopped or 1 teaspoon dry
2 cups cheese (gouda, cheddar, or any combo)
croutons or chopped almonds to taste

Directions:

1. Heat oven to 350 degrees.
2. Boil pasta in a large pot until al-dente.
3. Meanwhile, in a medium glass measuring cup, measure flour and butter. Microwave about 1-2 minutes until golden brown.
4. Slowly stir in milk and continue microwaving until thickened. Stir in spices and herbs.
5. Mix drained noodles, sauce, and cheese and put in a greased casserole dish. Bake about 20 minutes.
6. Top with croutons or chopped almonds in the last 5 minutes.

Nutrition Facts (per serving)
Calories 424 Carbohydrates 36 g
Protein 22 g Sodium 479 mg
Potassium 237 mg Phosphorus 428 mg

TURKEY PAPRIKASH

Ingredients:
Based on 4-5 servings per recipe.
1 onion, sliced
1/2 cup mushrooms
3 tablespoons butter or margarine
2 tablespoons flour
2 teaspoons paprika
1 cup low sodium turkey or chicken broth
2 egg yolks, slightly beaten
1 cup sour cream
2 cups diced cooked turkey
1/2 cup per person cooked noodles (poppy seed noodles optional) or cooked rice

2 tablespoons butter
1 teaspoon poppy seeds

Directions:

1. In saucepan, cook onion and mushrooms in butter until tender.
2. Blend in flour, paprika, and salt; add broth.
3. Cook and stir until mixture thickens and bubbles; cook 1 minute more.
4. Stir a small amount of hot mixture into egg yolks; return to hot mixture.
5. Cook over low heat for 1 minute more.
6. Stir in sour cream until blended.
7. Add turkey.
8. Heat slowly just until hot.
9. Serve over noodles or rice.
10. Toss with 2 tablespoons melted butter and 1 teaspoon poppy seeds.

Nutrition Facts (per serving)
Calories 519 Carbohydrates tbd
Protein 34,5 g Sodium 484 mg
Potassium 481 mg Phosphorus 356 mg

SPECIAL PIZZA

Ingredients:
Yield: 10 slices Serving size: 1 slice (5 ½" x 3" x ¼")
For crust:
2 cups all-purpose flour
1 teaspoon active dry yeast
1 tablespoon granulated sugar
1 cup water
2 tablespoons vegetable shortening

Directions:

1. In a large mixing bowl, combine flour, yeast and sugar.
2. Add shortening to dry ingredients; mix together using a fork.
3. Add water in small quantities while mixing with the fork until the mixture follows fork around the bowl.
4. Cover dough; allow it to rest for about 15 minutes.

Ingredients for pizza:
½ pound lean ground beef, turkey or chicken
½ teaspoon italian seasoning
½ teaspoon onion powder
½ teaspoon garlic powder
¼ cup tomato paste
1 teaspoon chili powder
1 teaspoon italian seasoning
½ cup water vegetable oil
4 ounces reduced fat sharp cheddar cheese, grated
½ cup diced green peppers
½ cup diced onions

Directions:

1. Preheat oven to 425°F.
2. In a frying pan, sauté ground meat. Add italianseasoning, onion powder and garlic powder; continue stirring until meat is browned.
3. Place meat on paper towels to drain.
4. In a bowl, prepare the sauce by mixing the tomato paste, chili powder, italian seasoning and water. Set aside.
5. After dough has rested, oil pizza pan and fingers. Spread dough evenly on pan.
6. Pour sauce evenly over pizza dough; sprinkle with ½ cup of cheese.
7. Cook in preheated oven for 15-20 minutes.
8. Remove from oven; add ground beef, remaining cheese, green peppers and onions. Return to oven for an additional 10 minutes. Serve hot.

Nutrition Facts (per serving)
Calories 196 Carbohydrates 24 g
Protein 11 g Sodium 144 mg
Potassium 188 mg Phosphorus 31 mg

BEEF AND BELL PEPPER PIZZA

Ingredients:
Yield: 6 portions Serving size: 1 slice (1/6 pizza)
1-1/4 teaspoons dry yeast
1-1/2 cups warm water
2 tablespoons olive oil
1 tablespoon sugar
2 cups all-purpose flour
3 ounces low-sodium tomato paste
1/4 teaspoon garlic powder
2 tablespoons Italian seasoning
1/4 cup onion
1/4 cup green bell pepper
1/2 pound ground beef
1/4 teaspoon black pepper
1/4 teaspoon crushed red pepper
6 ounces shredded mozzarella cheese

Directions:
1. Preheat oven to 425° F.
2. Dissolve yeast in 1 cup warm water. Stir in 1 tablespoon olive oil, sugar and flour to make dough. Place in a greased bowl, cover and set aside.
3. Combine tomato paste, 1/2 cup water, garlic powder, Italian seasoning and remaining oil in a small saucepan and simmer for 5 minutes.
4. Chop onion and bell pepper.
5. Brown meat with black pepper and crushed red pepper in a skillet. Drain off fat. Add onion and green pepper.

6. Spray a pizza pan or a 17" x 14" baking sheet with nonstick cooking spray . Press dough onto pan or sheet. Spread sauce, meat mixture and cheese over dough. Bake for 20 minutes or until dough and cheese are golden brown.
7. Cut into 6 slices.

Helpful hints:
1/2 package dry yeast equals 1-1/4 teaspoons.
Each pizza slice has only 1 ounce of cheese to keep phosphorus low.

Nutrition Facts (per serving)
Calories 402 Carbohydrates 38 g
Protein 22 g Sodium 150 mg
Potassium 352 mg Phosphorus 230 mg

DESSERT PIZZA

Ingredients:
Based on 8 servings per recipe.
1/2-1 cup part-skim ricotta cheese
2 cups canned peaches or fresh sliced strawberry
1/4-1/2 cup apricot jam or other light colored jam
5 tablespoons powdered sugar, divided
2 tablespoons warm jelly or preserves
1/4 cup chocolate chips
1 - 12 inch precooked pizza crust

Directions:
1. Preheat oven to 425 degrees.
2. Strain ricotta with cheesecloth or use coffee filter.
3. Drain peaches in colander and melt jam in microwave 30 seconds.
4. Brush jam on crust.

5. Mix ricotta and 3 tablespoons powdered sugar; spread on crust.
6. Top ricotta with peach or strawberry slices and sprinkle with remaining powdered sugar and chocolate chips.
7. Bake for 10-12 minutes.

Nutrition Facts (per serving)
Calories 288 Carbohydrates 49 g
Protein 8 g Sodium 166 mg
Potassium 98 mg Phosphorus 47 mg

MEDITERRANEAN PIZZA

Ingredients:
Based on 12 servings per recipe.
1 crust, 2 pitas ready made pizza dough or large pitas
1 tablespoon olive oil
2 garlic cloves, sliced thinly
1 roma tomato, sliced
10 basil leaves, thinly sliced
3 ounces goat cheese, or ricotta
Directions:
1. Preheat oven to 450 degrees.
2. Coat pizza crust with olive oil.
3. Arrange garlic slices evenly across the crust.
4. Cover garlic with tomato slices.
5. Sprinkle basil evenly over pizza then top with goat cheese.
6. Bake in oven for 10-15 minutes or as otherwise directed by crust package intructions.

Nutrition Facts (per serving)
Calories 176 Carbohydrates 18 g
Protein 7 g Sodium 240 mg
Potassium 86 mg Phosphorus 90 mg

ENGLISH MUFFIN PIZZA

Ingredients:
Yield: 1 serving Serving size: 2 pizzas
¼ cup pizza sauce
2 tablespoons shredded mozzarella cheese
Directions:
1. Toast english muffins.
2. Spread pizza sauce evenly on muffin halves.
3. Sprinkle cheese and add toppings.
4. Place the muffin halves on tray and put into toaster oven, set on broil.
5. Broil for about 5 minutes, watching carefully to remove when cheese is golden and melted.

Nutrition Facts (per serving)
Calories 253 Carbohydrates 33 g
Protein 13 g Sodium 529 mg
Potassium 324 mg Phosphorus 254 mg

BBQ RUB FOR PORK OR CHICKEN

Ingredients:
Based on 4 servings per recipe.
1 tablespoon brown sugar
1 teaspoon smoked paprika
1 teaspoon chili powder
1 teaspoon garlic, granulated
1 teaspoon onion powder
1 teaspoon cumin
1/4 teaspoon dry mustard powder
1/8 teaspoon allspice
1/8 teaspoon ground red pepper (optional)
Directions:

1. In a bowl, blend all ingredients together thoroughly.
2. Rub on pork or chicken before cooking.

Nutrition Facts (per serving)
Calories 20 Carbohydrates 4 g
Protein 0 g Sodium 9 mg
Potassium 34 mg Phosphorus 7 mg

FIRE AND ICE WATERMELON SALSA

Ingredients:
Based on 6 servings per recipe.
3 cups watermelon, chopped
1 cup green bell pepper, chopped
2 tablespoons lime juice
1 tablespoon cilantro, chopped
1 tablespoon green onion, chopped
2 medium jalapeño, seeded and minced
1 garlic clove, crushed

Directions:
1. Combine all ingredients, mix well.
2. Refrigerate for at least one hour before serving.
3. This is great as a dip or as a sauce for chicken or fish.

Nutrition Facts (per serving)
Calories 30 Carbohydrates 7 g
Protein 1 g Sodium 2 mg
Potassium 128 mg Phosphorus 14 mg

TABBOULEH

Ingredients:
Based on 8 servings per recipe.
1 cup bulgur wheat
1 cup warm water
1 tomato, peeled & chopped
1/2 medium cucumber, seeded & chopped
1/2 cup parsley, chopped
2 tablespoons green onion, finely chopped
1 tablespoon fresh mint, finely chopped
1/8 teaspoon pepper
3 tablespoons vegetable or olive oil

Directions:
1. In a bowl, combine bulgur and warm water.
2. Let stand for 30 minutes.
3. Stir in tomato, cucumber, parsley, green onion, mint, and pepper.
4. Combine oil and lemon juice.
5. Toss with the bulgur mixture.
6. Cover and chill.
7. Serve in a lettuce-lined bowl with yogurt, if desired.

Nutrition Facts (per serving)
Calories 115 Carbohydrates 15 g
Protein 3 g Sodium 7 mg
Potassium 180 mg Phosphorus 66 mg

ITALIAN DRESSING

Ingredients:
Yield: 16 serving Serving size: 2 tablespoons
1 tablespoon dried parsley
1/4 teaspoon ground oregano
1/2 teaspoon ground thyme
1/4 teaspoon ground marjoram
1/2 teaspoon ground celery seeds
1/4 teaspoon garlic powder
1 teaspoon granulated sugar
1/8 teaspoon salt
1 pinch black pepper

1/2 cup red wine vinegar
1/2 cup extra virgin olive oil

Directions:
1. Mix seasonings together.
2. Add to vinegar and oil.
3. Shake well to mix.

Helpful hints:
Homemade salad dressings keep well in the refrigerator for several weeks.
For variety try different oils, including flavored or spicy oils.

Nutrition Facts (per serving)
Calories 65 Carbohydrates 1 g
Protein 0 g Sodium 18 mg
Potassium 10 mg Phosphorus 1 mg

GREEN GARDEN SALAD

Ingredients:
Yield: 6 cups Serving size: 1 cup
4 cups red leaf or other lettuce, shredded
1 carrot, sliced 2 celery stalks, sliced
2 cucumbers, sliced 2 radishes, sliced
1 large bell pepper, diced or sliced into rings

Directions:
1. Combine vegetables in a large bowl and toss.
2. May serve with your favorite salad dressing.

Nutrition Facts (per serving)
Calories 30 Carbohydrates 4 g
Protein 1 g Sodium 20 mg
Potassium 215 mg Phosphorus 29 mg

BERRY WILD RICE SALAD

Ingredients:
Based on Nutrition facts estimated for 8 servings servings per recipe.
1 cup uncooked wild rice
2 cups water
1 cup collard greens, lightly steamed
1/2 cup onion, chopped
2 1/2 cups mixed berries (raspberry, blackberry, etc)
1/4 cup blueberries
2 tablespoons lemon juice
1/4 cup fresh mint, chopped
1 tablespoon olive oil
1/2 cup fat free or reduced fat sour cream

Directions:
1. Place rice and water in a large saucepan.
2. Bring to a boil, reduce heat to low and simmer covered for about 45-55 minutes, or until most of the liquid is absorbed.
3. Empty rice into a large mixing bowl and add steamed greens, onion, and berries.
4. Mix well.
5. In a blender or food processor, puree all dressing ingredients except sour cream until it is well blended, adding more liquid if necessary.
6. Slowly whisk in sour cream until well mixed.
7. Pour dressing over rice salad and toss to coat.
8. Serve immediately or store covered in the refrigerator for later use.

Nutrition Facts (per serving)
Calories 155 Carbohydrates 31 g
Protein 5 g Sodium 21 mg

Potassium 214 mg Phosphorus 98 mg

RASPBERRY VINAIGRETTE

Ingredients:
Based on 4-6 servings per recipe.
1/2 cup raspberry vinegar
1/4 cup oil
1 teaspoon dijon mustard
1 tablespoon sugar
1/4 cup mint leaves, chopped
Directions:
1. Whisk all ingredients together in small bowl.
2. Serve.

Nutrition Facts (per serving)
Calories 94 Carbohydrates 3 g
Protein 0 g Sodium 21 mg
Potassium 14 mg Phosphorus 2 mg

LEMON CURRY CHICKEN SALAD

Ingredients:
Based on 4 servings per recipe.
1/4 cup vegetable oil
1/4 cup frozen lemonade concentrate, thawed
1/4 teaspoon ground ginger
1/4 teaspoon curry powder
1/8 teaspoon garlic powder
1 1/2 cups chicken, cooked and diced
1 1/2 cups grapes, halved
1/2 cup celery, sliced
Directions:
1. In a large bowl, whisk together oil, lemonade concentrate, and spices.

2. Add remaining ingredients and toss lightly.
3. Chill at least an hour.

Nutrition Facts (per serving)
Calories 276 Carbohydrates 15 g
Protein 15 g Sodium 46 mg
Potassium 221 mg Phosphorus 82 mg

SUNSHINE SALAD

Ingredients:
Yield: 6-9 servings Serving size: 6 large or 9 small squares
1 package (3-ounces) lemon-flavored gelatin
1 cup boiling water
½ cup cold water
1 can (9-ounces)crushed pineapple, canned in its own juice
⅛ teaspoon salt
2 medium carrots mayonnaise for topping
Directions:
1. Empty gelatin packet into a small bowl.
2. Pour in boiling water, stir until gelatin is dissolved.
3. Stir in cold water, crushed pineapple and salt.
4. Chill the mixture in refrigerator until gelatin starts to thicken.
5. While mixture is cooling, peel and grate carrots.
6. Stir carrots into gelatin.
7. Pour into a square pan, (8" x 8" x 2"). Chill in refrigerator until firm.
8. Cut in squares. Lift out carefully and

serve on crisp lettuce leaves. Top with mayonnaise.

Nutrition Facts (per serving)
Calories 61 Carbohydrates 15 g
Protein 1 g Sodium 64 mg
Potassium 119 mg Phosphorus 25 mg

THAI SALAD WITH CORN

Ingredients:
Based on 4-6 servings per recipe.
zest and juice of 2 limes
2 garlic cloves, minced
2-3 tablespoons Thai sweet chili sauce
1/2 cups sweet corn kernels
1/2 red onion, chopped
1/2 cup, chopped cilantro
1/2 head cabbage, shredded*
1/2 cup shredded carrot
*If using pre-shredded mix, use 3 cups
Directions:
1. Combine lime juice, zest, garlic, and sweet chili sauce in a small bowl and stir until well mixed. Set aside.
2. In a large bowl, combine remaining ingredients and toss until well mixed.
3. Drizzle sauce onto vegetable mix and combine until vegetable mix is well coated.
4. Serve immediately or chill for up to 24 hours.

Nutrition Facts (per serving)
Calories 61 Carbohydrates 14 g
Protein 2 g Sodium 84 mg
Potassium 162 mg Phosphorus 15 mg

PASTA SALAD WITH ROASTED RED PEPPER SAUCE

Ingredients:
Based on 8 servings per recipe.
2 tablespoons mayonnaise
8 leaves fresh basil
1 clove fresh garlic
2 tablespoons balsamic vinegar
2 small roasted red bell peppers (canned ok)
1 (16 ounce) package penne pasta
1 tablespoon olive oil
1 large sweet yellow onion, sliced
Directions:
1. Puree mayonnaise, basil, garlic, vinegar, and peppers together in a food processor or blender.
2. Cook pasta according to package directions, rinse with cold water and set aside.
3. Heat oil in a medium frying pan over medium heat.
4. Add sliced onion and saute until the onion caramelizes (turns soft and lightly brown).
5. Combine pasta, caramelized onions and sauce in a large bowl.
6. Pasta salad may be eaten immediately or it may be kept in the refrigerator for up to 3 days.

Nutrition Facts (per serving)
Calories 265 Carbohydrates 47 g
Protein 8 g Sodium 85 mg
Potassium 150 mg Phosphorus 91 mg

CHICKEN N' ORANGE SALAD SANDWICH

Ingredients:
Based on 6 servings per recipe.
1 cup chopped cooked chicken
1/2 cup celery, diced
1/2 cup green pepper, chopped
1/4 cup onion, finely sliced
1 cup Mandarin oranges
1/3 cup mayonnaise
Directions:
1. Toss chicken, celery, green pepper, and onion to mix.
2. Add mandarin oranges and mayonnaise.
3. Mix gently.
4. Serve on bread.

Nutrition Facts (per serving)
Calories 162 Carbohydrates 6 g
Protein 12 g Sodium 93 mg
Potassium 241 mg Phosphorus 106 mg

MACARONI SALADS

Ingredients:
3 cups macaroni, cooked
¼ cup pimentos
½ cup onion, chopped
½ cup green pepper, chopped
3 hard boiled, shelled eggs, chopped
½ cup mayonnaise
½ cupcelery, chopped
1 teaspoon dry mustard
paprika
black pepper
Directions:

1. Rinse cooked macaroni under cold water; drain well.
2. Combine macaroni with remaining ingredients except paprika and black pepper. Mix well.
3. Sprinkle with paprika and black pepper.
4. Chill and serve.

Nutrition Facts (per serving)
Calories 223 Carbohydrates 18 g
Protein 6 g Sodium 103 mg
Potassium 106 mg Phosphorus 74 mg

POTATO SALAD

Ingredients:
2 tbsp. sweet pickle relish
1 tps. celery seed
1/3 cup chopped onion
2 cups leached potatoes
1/3 cup diced raw celery
paparika for garnish
1/4 cup reduced fat mayonnaise
Directions:
1. Boil leached water potatoes (use 5 cups water for each cup of potatoes), until tender but not mushy.
2. In a bowl, mix together relish onions, celery, mayo and celery seed. Toss in potatoes.
3. Sprinkle with paparika. Refrigerate to blend flavors for at least one hour.
Leaching instructions: Peel, cut into small pieces, exposing as much surface area as possible. Rinse in warm water for a few seconds. Place potatoes in a large container and add large amount of tap water (use 10 cups of water for each cup

of potatoes). Soak for 2-4 hours at room temperatue. Drain and rinse the leached potatoes.

Nutrition Facts (per serving)
Carbohydrates 19 g Protein 2 g
Sodium 206 mg Potassium 174 mg
Phosphorus 45 mg

APPLE RICE SALAD

Ingredients:
Based on 4 servings per recipe.
2 tablespoons balsamic vinegar
1 tablespoon olive oil
2 teaspoons honey
2 teaspoons brown or dijon mustard
1 tablespoon orange peel, finely shredded
1/4 teaspoon garlic powder
2 cups cooked rice (any kind), chilled
2 cups (about 2 medium) apples, chopped
1 cup celery, thinly sliced
2 tablespoons unsalted sunflower seeds, shelled
Directions:
1. In a small bowl, combine the vinegar, olive oil, honey, mustard, orange peel, and garlic powder. Mix well and set aside.
2. In a large bowl, combine rice, apples, celery, and sunflower seeds. Toss until well mixed.
3. Drizzle the dressing over the rice salad mixture and toss until salad is well coated.
4. Serve immediately or cover and refrigerate for up to 24 hours.

Nutrition Facts (per serving)
Calories 238 Carbohydrates 42 g
Protein 4 g Sodium 227 mg
Potassium 238 mg Phosphorus 82 mg

SHRIMP SALAD

Ingredients:
Yield: 4 servings Serving size: ½ cup
1 pound shrimp, boiled, chopped and deveined
1 hard boiled egg, chopped
1 tablespoon celery, chopped
1 tablespoon green pepper, chopped
1 tablespoon onion, chopped
2 tablespoons mayonnaise
1 teaspoon lemon juice
½ teaspoon chili powder
⅛ teaspoon Tabasco® or hot sauce
½ teaspoon dry mustard lettuce, chopped or shredded (optional)
Directions:
1. Combine all ingredients except lettuce in a mixing bowl; mix well.
2. Chill in refrigerator for 30 minutes.
3. Serve as a salad over a bed of lettuce, if desired, or serve on a sandwich.

Nutrition Facts (per serving)
Calories 157 Carbohydrates 1 g
Protein 26 g Sodium 232 mg
Potassium 233 mg Phosphorus 263 mg

CHICKEN SALAD DELIGHT

Ingredients:
Yield: 5 servings Serving size: ¾ cup
2 cups chicken, diced
⅓ cup celery, chopped
¼ cup fresh onion, chopped
¼ cup fresh green pepper, chopped
1 teaspoon parsley, dried (optional)
1 tablespoon lemon juice
¼ teaspoon black pepper
1 teaspoon dry mustard
½ cup mayonnaise

Directions:
1. Combine chicken, celery, onion, green pepper, parsley and toss with lemon juice.
2. In a bowl, combine black pepper, mustard, and mayonnaise. Add to chicken mixture, mixing thoroughly.

Nutrition Facts (per serving)
Calories 181 Carbohydrates 3 g
Protein 18 g Sodium 239 mg
Potassium 205 mg Phosphorus 149 mg

CHICKEN VEGETABLE SALAD

Ingredients:
Yield: 4 servings Serving size: ½ cup
1 ½ cups cooked chicken, diced
½ cup green pepper, finely chopped
½ cup celery, finely diced
½ cup onions, finely chopped
3 tablespoons pimentos, diced
½ cup salad dressing or light mayonnaise
1 tablespoon lemon juice

Directions:
1. In a large bowl, combine chicken, green pepper, celery, onions and pimentos.
2. In a small bowl, mix mayonnaise and lemon juice. Pour over chicken mixture.
3. Mix well, cover and chill.
4. Serve in a lettuce cups.

Nutrition Facts (per serving)
Calories 221 Carbohydrates 15 g
Protein 18 g Sodium 245 mg
Potassium 230 mg Phosphorus 143 mg

SALT-FREE SWEET BROWN MUSTARD

Ingredients:
Yield: 1 ½ cups Serving size: 1 tablespoon
2 teaspoons cornstarch
1 cup cider vinegar
½ cup dry mustard
½ cup light brown sugar
½ teaspoon white pepper (or black pepper)

Directions:
1. Dissolve cornstarch in small amount of vinegar.
2. Heat remaining vinegar; add mustard, sugar, and pepper. Stir until dissolved.
3. When hot, add cornstarch and cook until thick. Remove from heat.
4. Cover the mixture and let stand at room temperature for 24 hours to develop flavor.

Nutrition Facts (per serving)
Calories 27 Carbohydrates 4 g
Protein 0 g Sodium 2 mg
Potassium 27 mg Phosphorus 18 mg

LOW SALT GUACAMOLE

Ingredients:
Based on 16 servings per recipe.
1 medium avocado
1 tablespoon lemon juice
3 tablespoons sour cream (light or regular)
1 small tomato, chopped
1 onion, chopped
1/8 teaspoon chili powder or more for extra spice
Directions:
1. Crush avocado and lemon juice together with fork.
2. When softened add in the sour cream and crush some more.
3. Add in the tomato, onion, and chili powder and stir until evenly distributed.
4. Chill and serve with no salt or low salt tortilla chips.

Nutrition Facts (per serving)
Calories 25 Carbohydrates 2 g
Protein tbd Sodium 4 mg
Potassium 89 mg Phosphorus 3 mg

RELISH

Ingredients:
Yield: 2 ¼ cups Serving size: 1 tablespoon
2 lemons, peeled and quartered
1 large onion
½ medium green pepper
2 cups sliced celery
¼ cup parsley (optional)
½ cup sugar
¼ teaspoon ground mustard

⅛ teaspoon allspice
1 teaspoon celery seed
Directions:
1. Chop first five ingredients. Stir in sugar and spices.
2. Cover and place in refrigerator for several hours or overnight to blend flavors.

Nutrition Facts (per serving)
Calories 8 Carbohydrates 2 g
Protein 0 g Sodium 8 mg
Potassium 31 mg Phosphorus 9 mg

SOUR CREAM DILL SAUCE

Ingredients:
Based on 8 servings per recipe.
1- 8 ounce container sour cream
2 tablespoons fresh dill, chopped
2 tablespoons fresh lemon juice
1 clove garlic, minced
Directions:
1. Mix ingredients together in a food processor or blender until smooth.
2. Refrigerate overnight.
3. Serve over seafood or fresh vegetables.

Nutrition Facts (per serving)
Calories 62 Carbohydrates 2 g
Protein 1 g Sodium 15 mg
Potassium 48 mg Phosphorus 25 mg

LOW SALT KETCHUP

Ingredients:
Based on 64 servings per recipe.

3/4 cup onion, chopped
1/2 cup cider vinegar
1/3 cup sugar
1 tablespoon molasses
2 teaspoons dry mustard
1/2 teaspoon celery seed
1/4 teaspoon ground cinnamon
1/4 teaspoon cloves
1/4 teaspoon dried basil
1/4 teaspoon dried tarragon
1/4 teaspoon pepper
1 clove garlic, minced
1 cup water
2 (6-oz.) can tomato paste

Directions:

1. Place all ingredients except water and tomato paste in a blender or food processor, blend until smooth.
2. Pour mixture into a Dutch oven or large sauce pan.
3. Stir in 3 cups water and two 6-oz. cans tomato paste.
4. Simmer, uncovered, about 35 minutes or until mixture is reduced to half its original amount, stirring occasionally.
5. Pour into jars and store in refrigerator for up to 1 month. Or pour into 1-cup freezer containers; seal, label, and freeze for up to 10 months. Makes 5 cups.

Nutrition Facts (per serving)
Calories 12 Carbohydrates 3 g
Protein 0 g Sodium 17 mg
Potassium 62 mg Phosphorus 1 mg

SIMPLE WHITE SAUCE

Ingredients:
Based on 4 servings per recipe.
2 tablespoons flour
2 tablespoons margarine or Unsalted butter
1 cup heavy cream
1/4 teaspoon dry mustard
1/4 teaspoon paprika
1/2 teaspoon fresh or 1 teaspoon dried parsley, basil, or other herb

Directions:
1. Mix flour and margarine or butter together in a 2 cup glass measuring cup or small microwave-safe bowl.
2. Microwave for 30 seconds, stir, microwave another 30 seconds.
3. Add cream and spices and stir.
4. Microwave 1 minute, stir again.
5. Microwave 1 minute.
6. If not thickened, add 1 more minute.

Nutrition Facts (per serving)
Calories 273 Carbohydrates 5 g
Protein 2 g Sodium 25 mg
Potassium 54 mg Phosphorus 43 mg

SPICY BARBECUE SAUCE

Ingredients:
Yield: 1 ½ cup Serving size: 1 tablespoon
¼ cup dark corn syrup
¼ cup red wine vinegar
¼ cup onion, chopped
1 cup water
2 teaspoons dry mustard
2 tablespoons tomato paste

1 teaspoon Tabasco® pepper sauce
2 tablespoons vegetable oil
1 tablespoon all purpose flour
1 teaspoon Mrs. Dash® (of your choice)

Directions:
1. Mix all ingredients together except vegetable oil and flour in a sauce pan.
2. Mix vegetable oil and flour together in separate container to make paste.
3. Add to sauce pan, cook on low heat until desired thickness is reached.
4. Pour or brush on baked or grilled meats.

Nutrition Facts (per serving)
Calories 28 Carbohydrates 2 g
Protein 0 g Sodium 28 mg
Potassium 34 mg Phosphorus 7 mg

HOMEMADE LOW-SODIUM SOY SAUCE

Ingredients:
Based on 32 servings per recipe.
5 packets Herb-Ox Sodium Free Boullion, beef or chicken flavor
6 tablespoons cider or balsamic vinegar
4-5 tablespoons molasses
2 cups boiling water
1/4 teaspoon black pepper
1/4 teaspoon powdered ginger
1/4 teaspoon garlic powder
2 tablespoons Kikkoman Less Sodium Soy Sauce

Directions:
1. Mix all ingredients.
2. Pour into bottle and store in refrigerator. Keeps indefinitel

Nutrition Facts (per serving)
Calories 10 Carbohydrates 2 g
Protein 0 g Sodium 38 mg
Potassium 113 mg Phosphorus 3 mg

ALFREDO SAUCE

Ingredients:
Based on 8 servings per recipe.
1/4 cup olive oil
3 tablespoons all-purpose flour
1 clove garlic, minced
2 cups rice milk
4 ounces cream cheese
1/3 cup shredded Parmesan cheese
1/4 teaspoon ground nutmeg
1 tablespoon lemon juice

Directions:
1. Heat olive oil in a large skillet over medium heat. Add flour and whisk to make a paste then add minced garlic.
2. Slowly add rice milk, whisking constantly to prevent lumps. Let mixture come to a boil and thicken.
3. Add cream cheese and mix well. Remove from heat.
4. Add 1/3 cup Parmesan cheese, nutmeg, and lemon juice. Mix well.
5. Serve over pasta, chicken, steamed vegetables, etc.

Nutrition Facts (per serving)
Calories 173 Carbohydrates 9 g
Protein 3 g Sodium 142 mg
Potassium 32 mg Phosphorus 75 mg

PICO DE GALLO

Ingredients:
Yield: 8 servings Serving size: 1/4 c
3–6 garlic cloves (Depending on preference)
~1 cup jicama
1/2 sweet onion or purple onion
1/4 c lime juice or to taste
pinch of salt
1 tbsp sugar

Directions:
Add all ingredients to food processor and pulse to make salsa.

Nutrition Facts (per serving)
Calories 33 Carbohydrates 7,4 g
Protein 1 g Sodium 294 mg
Potassium 144 mg Phosphorus 19 mg

STEAMED ASPARAGUS

Ingredients:
Yield: 4 servings Serving size: 3 spears
1 tablespoon lemon juice
2 tablespoons margarine, melted (unsalted)
2 cups water
12 fresh asparagus spears

Directions:
1. Add lemon juice to margarine; set aside.
2. Bring water to a boil in bottom of steamer.
3. Place asparagus in steamer over boiling water.
4. Steam for 2 minutes after asparagus turns bright green.
5. Remove and pour margarine with lemon juice over asparagus. Serve.

Nutrition Facts (per serving)
Calories 62 Carbohydrates 3 g
Protein 1 g Sodium 1 mg
Potassium 123 mg Phosphorus 32 mg

ROASTED GREEN BEANS AND SWEET ONION

Ingredients:
Based on 8 servings per recipe.
1 pound sweet onions, cut into 1/2 pieces
2 tablespoons olive oil
2/3 pound green beans
2 tablespoons balsamic vinegar

Directions:
1. Preheat oven to 375 degrees.
2. Place onions in a large roasting pan.
3. Drizzle onions with olive oil and toss to coat evenly.
4. Place in oven and roast for 30 minutes, turning about every 10 minutes.
5. Add green beans to the onions and roast for another 10 minutes.
6. Add balsamic vinegar and cook in oven for another 2 to 5 minute.

Nutrition Facts (per serving)
Calories 63 Carbohydrates 7 g
Protein 1 g Sodium 6 mg
Potassium 161 mg Phosphorus 15 mg

WILD RICE STUFFING

Ingredients:
Based on 8-10 servings per recipe.
2 cups uncooked wild rice
4 cups low sodium turkey, chicken or mushroom broth
2 cups mushrooms, sliced
1 onion, chopped
1 cup dried apricots, chopped
1 cup dried cherries, chopped
1/4 cup butter or margarine
1 cup water chestnuts, diced
1 cup shelled pistachio nuts
1/4 cup fresh or 1 teaspoon dried thyme
1/4 cup fresh or 1 teaspoon dried tarragon

Directions:
1. Cook 2 cups wild rice in low sodium turkey, chicken, or mushroom broth.
2. Preheat oven to 350 degrees.
3. Saute mushrooms, onion, apricots, cherries in butter.
4. Add water chestnuts, pistachios and rice. Cook, stirring, for about 5 minutes.
5. Add herbs and place in greased baking dish and bake about 30 minutes.
6. Great side dish to turkey at Thanksgiving or with a roast chicken. You can double or triple the recipe and freeze it, it keeps well for months.

Nutrition Facts (per serving)
Calories 297 Carbohydrates 46 g
Protein 7 g Sodium 10 mg
Potassium 611 mg Phosphorus 146 mg

FRIED ONION RINGS

Ingredients:
Yield: 10 servings Serving size: 7 rings
¾ cup plain cornmeal
¼ cup all-purpose flour
1 teaspoon sugar 4 medium onions
1 egg, beaten
¼ cup water
½ cup vegetable oil for frying

Directions:
1. Mix cornmeal, flour and sugar together; set aside.
2. Peel onions, and cut crosswise about ¼" thick. Separate into rings.
3. Mix beaten egg and water.
4. Dip rings in egg wash, then into cornmeal mixture.
5. Fry rings for 3-5 minutes in hot vegetable oil, turning until brown.
6. Drain on paper towel. Serve hot.

Nutrition Facts (per serving)
Calories 162 Carbohydrates 14 g
Protein 2 g Sodium 11 mg
Potassium 99 mg Phosphorus 39 mg

HEARTY MASHED POTATOES

Ingredients:
Based on 8 servings per recipe.
2 pounds potatoes
1/4 cup unsalted butter
1/2 cup milk

Directions:
1. Peel potatoes and slice thinly, about 1/8 inch thick.
2. Rinse well.

3. Place sliced potatoes in a large pot of water so that there is at least 4 times more water than potatoes (about 9 quarts of water).

4. Soak for at least 1 hour (If you are not concerned with your potassium levels you may skip the soaking).

5. Drain and rinse soaked potatoes.

6. Place soaked potatoes in a large stockpot.

7. Fill rest of pot with water.

8. Bring to a boil then boil for 10 minutes.

9. Discard water.

10. Transfer boiled potatoes to a large mixing bowl.

11. Mash lightly with a potato masher or use a hand mixer on low speed until just mashed.

12. Mix in butter.

13. Add milk slowly until desired consistency is reached. Be careful not to over mash or the potatoes may develop a glue-like consistency.

Nutrition Facts (per serving)
Calories 157 Carbohydrates 23 g
Protein 2 g Sodium 13 mg
Potassium 180 mg Phosphorus 61 mg

MARINATED VEGETABLES

Ingredients:
Yield: 15 servings Serving size: ½ cup
For marinade:
¾ cup vinegar
¾ cup sugar
1 tablespoon water black pepper, to taste
Ingredient for salad:
1 12-ounce can small english peas, drained

1 12-ounce can shoe peg corn*, drained
1 12-ounce jarpimento, drained
¾ cup onion, finely chopped
1 cup celery, finely chopped
Directions:
1. In a small saucepan, combine marinade ingredients, and bring to a boil. Cool completely.

2. Mix salad ingredients together.

3. Pour cooled marinade over vegetables and stir.

4. Place in a covered container and refrigerate overnight before serving.
Tip: if unable to find shoepeg corn substitute with white or yellow corn.

Nutrition Facts (per serving)
Calories 85 Carbohydrates 20 g
Protein 1 g Sodium 13 mg
Potassium 154 mg Phosphorus 39 mg

GREEN BEANS WITH HAZELNUTS AND DRIED CRANBERRIES

Ingredients:
Based on 8 servings per recipe.
1 1/2 pounds fresh (or frozen) green beans
1/2 cup hazelnuts
12 cups water
3 tablespoons olive oil
1/3 cup shallots, thinly sliced
1/2 cup dried cranberries
1/2 teaspoon lemon zest
Directions:
1. Preheat oven to 350 degrees.

2. Spread hazelnuts in a single layer on

a baking sheet. Bake at 350 degrees for 10-15 minutes or until the skins begin to split, turn once.

3. Transfer toasted nuts to a colander or dish, and rub briskly with a towel to remove the skins. Coarsely chop nuts.

4. Bring 12 cups of water to a boil in a large saucepan. Add beans, cook 4 minutes or until crisp-tender. Drain and plunge into ice water, drain. Pat beans dry.

5. Heat a large skillet over medium heat. Add oil to pan, swirl to coat. Add shallots, cook until lightly browned. Add beans, cook 3 minutes or until thoroughly heated, stirring occasionally. Add cranberries and hazelnuts, cook 1 minute. Sprinkle with lemon zest.

Nutrition Facts (per serving)
Calories 199 Carbohydrates 17 g
Protein 4 g Sodium 19 mg
Potassium 246 mg Phosphorus 73 mg

FRAGRANT & FLAVORFUL BASMATI RICE

Ingredients:
Based on 8 servings per recipe.
1 tablespoon unsalted butter
1/2 teaspoon ground turmeric
1/2 teaspoon ground coriander
1/2 teaspoon ground cardamom
1 clove garlic, minced
1 cup ghite basmati rice
1 2/3 cups low sodium chicken broth
Directions:
Heat butter in a large skillet over medium heat.

1. Add spices and garlic.
2. Saute for 1 minute.
3. Add rice and stir until coated with butter and spices.
4. Add chicken broth.
5. Bring to a boil, then reduce heat to medium-low.
6. Cover and simmer for 15 minutes

Nutrition Facts (per serving)
Calories 114 Carbohydrates 21 g
Protein 3 g Sodium 25 mg
Potassium 49 mg Phosphorus 17 mg

VEGETABLES & RICE

Ingredients:
Yield: 6 servings Serving size: ½ cup
2 ½ cups rice, cooked, salt-free
1 10-ounce package frozen green peas, cooked and drained
1 medium onion, chopped
¼ cup margarine, unsalted
1 tablespoon lemon juice
½ teaspoon thyme
2 tablespoons liquid smoke (optional)
Directions:
1. Sauté chopped onion in margarine until tender.
2. Add rice, green peas, lemon juice, thyme and liquid smoke.
3. Cook for 5 minutes.

Nutrition Facts (per serving)
Calories 194 Carbohydrates 26 g
Protein 4 g Sodium 32 mg
Potassium 99 mg Phosphorus 67 mg

KALE AND TURNIP GREENS

Ingredients:
Based on 12 (1/2 cup each) servings per recipe.
2 pounds kale
2 pounds turnip greens (mustard greens will work)
1/4 cup olive oil
2 onions, chopped
1 clove of garlic, minced
3 tomatoes, chopped

Directions:
1. Wash kale and greens thoroughly.
2. Heat olive oil in a large skillet.
3. Add onions and cook until soft.
4. Add garlic, then tomatoes.
5. Cook over medium-low heat uncovered for 5 minutes.
6. Meanwhile, chop the greens.
7. Lay greens over tomato mixture, cover with lid and cook for 15 minutes or until all greens are wilted.

Nutrition Facts (per serving)
Calories 60 Carbohydrates 8 g
Protein 2 g Sodium 33 mg
Potassium 335 mg Phosphorus 45 mg

BAKED YELLOW SQUASH

Ingredients:
Yield: 6 servings Serving size: ½ cup
2 tablespoons margarine or butter, melted
¾ teaspoon thyme
⅛ teaspoon black pepper
2 cans yellow squash, sliced
1 medium onion, chopped
1 small stalk celery, chopped
1 large bell pepper, chopped
1 tablespoon lemon juice

Directions:
1. Preheat oven to 350°F.
2. Sauté all ingredients except lemon juice in margarine. Cook until onions are translucent.
3. Add lemon juice.
4. Place sautéed mixture in a casserole dish.
5. Bake for approximately 30 minutes. Serve hot.

Nutrition Facts (per serving)
Calories 49 Carbohydrates 5 g
Protein 1 g Sodium 34 mg
Potassium 139 mg Phosphorus 25 mg

HONEY GLAZED CARROTS

Ingredients:
Based on 6 servings per recipe.
6 carrots, cut on bias
1 1/2 cups water
3 tablespoons sugar
1 tablespoon butter, cut into 4 pieces
2 tablespoons lemon juice pepper to tast

Directions:
1. Bring carrots, water and 1 tablespoon sugar to boil.
2. Cover and reduce heat, simmering about 5 minutes
3. Uncover and reduce 1-2 minutes.
4. Add butter and remaining sugar.
5. Stir for 3 minutes.
6. Remove and add lemon juice

Nutrition Facts (per serving)
Calories 108 Carbohydrates 20 g
Protein 1 g Sodium 75 mg
Potassium 256 mg Phosphorus 39 mg

ALMOST MASHED POTATOES

Ingredients:
Yield: 6 servings Serving size: 1/2 cup
6 cups cauliflower
4 ounces cream cheese
1 teaspoon garlic
1/2 teaspoon black pepper
Directions:
1. Cut the cauliflower into pieces and rinse with water.
2. Place the cauliflower pieces in a microwave safe dish, cover and cook on high for 8 to 10 minutes or until soft.
3. Drain off moisture from the cooked cauliflower.
4. Carefully place the hot cauliflower in a blender and blend until smooth.
5. Add the cream cheese, garlic and pepper. Blend to combine ingredients.
6. Remove mixture from the blender and serve hot.
Helpful hints:
One medium head cauliflower yields 6 cups.
Garlic powder may be substituted for the minced garlic.
Since cauliflower is bland like potatoes, this recipe tastes similar to mashed potatoes. The potassium content is 100 mg lower per serving.
To reduce fat content, use light cream cheese. Protein, sodium, potassium and phosphorus content will be slightly

higher.

Nutrition Facts (per serving)
Calories 94 Carbohydrates 6 g
Protein 3 g Sodium 76 mg
Potassium 198 mg Phosphorus 54 mg

FAVORITE GREEN BEANS

Ingredients:
Yield: 6 servings Serving size: ½ cup
2 cans whole green beans, drained and rinsed
1 small onion, chopped
½ cup fresh mushrooms, sliced
1 teaspoon paprika
¼ teaspoon coarse black pepper
1 ½ cups unsalted top cracker crumbs
4 tablespoons margarine, unsalted
Directions:
1. Preheat oven to 350°F.
2. Mix together green beans, onion, mushrooms, paprika and black pepper.
3. Place in a greased baking dish.
4. Top green bean mixture with cracker crumbs and margarine.
5. Bake for 30-35 minutes.

Nutrition Facts (per serving)
Calories 137 Carbohydrates 14 g
Protein 2 g Sodium 77 mg
Potassium 214 mg Phosphorus 38 mg

PURPLE AND GOLD THAI COLESLAW

Ingredients:
Based on 12 servings per recipe.

Dressing below:
5 tablespoons rice vinegar
5 tablespoons canola oil
1.5 tablespoons lite soy sauce
3 tablespoons brown sugar
2 tablespoons ginger, peeled and minced
1/2 tablespoon garlic, minced
5 tablespoons no salt peanut butter
Slaw below:
7 cups red cabbage
2 cups yellow pepper, sliced or chopped
bunch (~8) or ~3/4 cup green onions,
sliced
1/2 bunch fresh cilantro

Directions:
1. Combine the dressing ingredients in a small bowl.
2. Mix dressing well into the slaw mixture

Nutrition Facts (per serving)
Calories 140 Carbohydrates 10 g
Protein 3 g Sodium 79 mg
Potassium 228 mg Phosphorus 29 mg

PINEAPPLE COLESLAW

Ingredients:
Based on 4 servings per recipe.
2 cups shredded cabbage
1 - 8 ounce can crushed, unsweetened
pineapple, drained
1/4 cup onion, chopped
1 red apple, cubed
1 carrot, grated
1/4 cup miracle whip or mayonnaise

Directions:
1. Mix all ingredients together and chill for 1 hour before serving.

Nutrition Facts (per serving)
Calories 128 Carbohydrates 8 g
Protein 1 g Sodium 81 mg
Potassium 143 mg Phosphorus 14 mg

COLESLAW

Ingredients:
Yield: 4 servings Serving size: ½ cup
1 cup cabbage, shredded
2 tablespoons green pepper, chopped
¼ cup onion, chopped
¼ cup carrots, shredded
¼ cup mayonnaise
2 tablespoons vinegar
1 tablespoon sugar
½ teaspoon black pepper
½ teaspoon celery seed (optional)
⅛ teaspoon dill weeds (optional)

Directions:
1. Combine vegetables.
2. Blend mayonnaise, vinegar and seasonings.
3. Pour over vegetables and toss.

Nutrition Facts (per serving)
Calories 127 Carbohydrates 6 g
Protein 0 g Sodium 81 mg
Potassium 76 mg Phosphorus 14 mg

PULLED PORK BBQ STYLE

Ingredients:
Based on 10-12 servings per recipe.
1 cup low sodium ketchup
1 cup no-salt added tomato sauce
2/3 cup brown sugar

2/3 cup red wine vinegar
1/4 cup molasses
2 teaspoons liquid smoke
1/4 teaspoon garlic powder
1/4 teaspoon onion powder
1/4 teaspoon chili powder
1/2 teaspoon paprika
1/4 teaspoon celery seed
1/4 teaspoon cinnamon
1/4 teaspoon cayenne
1/2 teaspoon black pepper
4 pounds pork shoulder roast

Directions:

1. Mix all ingredients except pork in a bowl to make the BBQ sauce.
2. Place pork into the crock pot and pour the BBQ sauce over the pork.
3. Set on high heat for 6 hours or on low overnight.
4. Meat is done when it reaches 165 degrees.
5. Shred pork by pulling apart with two forks.
6. Serve on a hamburger bun, roll, or with rice.

Nutrition Facts (per serving)
Calories 403 Carbohydrates 24 g
Protein 27 g Sodium 90 mg
Potassium 652 mg Phosphorus 241 mg

SUMMER SALAD

Ingredients:
Based on 4 servings per recipe.
1 small head bibb or butter lettuce, torn
6-8 strawberries, sliced
1 (11 ounce) can mandarin oranges, chilled and drained

1 small purple onion, sliced in rings
1/4 cup toasted slivered almonds
1/4 cup parmesan cheese, shredded
1/4 cup olive oil
2 Tablespoons balsamic vinegar
1 teaspoon sugar
1/8 teaspoon pepper

Directions:

1. Combine salad ingredients in a large salad bowl.
2. Combine dressing ingredients: olive oil, balsamic vinegar, sugar, and pepper in a jar. Cover lightly and shake until mixed well.
3. Pour mixture over salad, toss gently to coat.
4. Serve immediately.

Nutrition Facts (per serving)
Calories 250 Carbohydrates 14 g
Protein 5 g Sodium 95 mg
Potassium 265 mg Phosphorus 104 mg

BEEF JERKY

Ingredients:
Based on 30 servings per recipe.
3 pounds flank steak or other lean meat
3/4 cup sodium reduced (lite) soy sauce
1/2 cup red wine
1/4 cup dark brown sugar
2 tablespoons liquid smoke
1 1/2 teaspoons Worcestershire sauce
2-3 drops Tabasco sauce
1 teaspoon garlic powder
1 teaspoon liquid pepper sauce

Directions:

1. Trim (or have the butcher trim) all fat from a 3 pound flank steak or any lean

meat.

2. Cut lengthwise, with the grain, into 30 long strips.

3. Place the strips in a glass dish.

4. mix all other ingredients together and pour over the beef.

5. Cover and refrigerate for at least 5 hours or overnight.

6. When you are ready to dry the meat, remove it from the marinade.

7. If you have a dehydrator, set it for 145 degrees and dry the meat for 5-20 hours.

8. If you are using the oven, preheat to 175 degrees.

9. Put wire racks on top of baking sheets and lay the strips so they are not overlapping .

10. Bake for 10-12 hours. The beef jerky should be dry and somewhat brittle when done.

Store your jerky in an airtight container or plastic bag. If you are keeping it for longer than a week, store it in the freezer.

Nutrition Facts (per serving)
Calories 100 Carbohydrates tbd
Protein 12 g Sodium 100 mg
Potassium 100 mg Phosphorus 190 mg

FRUIT OMELET

Ingredients:
Yield: 4 servings Serving size: ¼ omelet
2 cups frozen unsweetened strawberries, thawed
1 tablespoon sugar (optional)
4 eggs, separated
1 tablespoon lemon juice
1 tablespoon unsalted butter or margarine

Directions:
1. Preheat oven to 375ºF.

2. Sprinkle thawed strawberries with sugar; let stand.

3. Beat egg whites in a medium bowl until stiff.

4. Beat egg yolks and lemon juice in a separate bowl. Fold stifflybeaten egg whites into beaten yolks untilno yellow streaks remain.

5. Melt butter in a 10" skillet that is oven-safe. Pour egg mixture into skillet, tilting pan to coat sides. Cook over low heat 5 minutes.

6. When mixture is set on the bottom, cook in oven for 5 additional minutes.

7. Lift omelet onto heated plate. Spoon on strawberries. Cut into pie wedges. Serve hot.

Nutrition Facts (per serving)
Calories 198 Carbohydrates 24 g
Protein 8 g Sodium 125 mg
Potassium 430 mg Phosphorus 141 mg

HERBED OMELET

Ingredients:
Yield: 2 servings Serving size: ½ omelet
1 ½ teaspoons vegetable oil
1 tablespoon chopped onion
4 eggs
2 tablespoons water
¼ teaspoon basil
⅛ teaspoon tarragon
¼ teaspoon parsley (optional)
Directions:

1. Beat eggs; add water and spices.
2. Heat oil in 8" frying pan over medium heat, add onions and sauté. Remove from pan.
3. Pour mixture into heated frying pan over medium heat.
4. As the omelet sets, lift with a spatula to let the uncooked portion of the omelet flow to the bottom.
5. When the omelet is completely set, add the sautéed onion to the top of the omelet and remove from pan to a serving dish.

Nutrition Facts (per serving)
Calories 195 Carbohydrates 0 g
Protein 14 g Sodium 157 mg
Potassium 157 mg Phosphorus 214 mg

COLESLAW WITH A KICK

Ingredients:
Based on 10 servings per recipe.
1 cup mayonnaise
1 tablespoon horseradish
2 teaspoons cider vinegar
3 tablespoons granulated sugar
2 teaspoons fresh dill, chopped
1 (1 pound) bag coleslaw mix with carrots
Directions:
1. In a large bowl, whisk together the mayonnaise, horseradish, vinegar, sugar and dill.
2. Stir in coleslaw mix until well blended.
3. Chill at least 1 hour. Will taste best if chilled overnight.

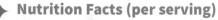

Nutrition Facts (per serving)
Calories 107 Carbohydrates 8 g
Protein 0 g Sodium 170 mg
Potassium 117 mg Phosphorus 11 mg

YELLOW SQUASH & GREEN ONIONS

Ingredients:
Yield: 3 servings Serving size: ½ cup
2 cups yellow straight neck or crook neck squash, washed and sliced
2 tablespoons butter or margarine
1 cup green onion, chopped
1 teaspoon black pepper
Directions:
1. Boil squash slices for 15 minutes or until tender; drain.
2. In frying pan, melt butter. Sauté onions until tender.
3. Stir in squash and black pepper.
4. Cover and allow to simmer on low heat for about 5 minutes. Serve hot.

Nutrition Facts (per serving)
Calories 87 Carbohydrates 4 g
Protein 0 g Sodium 170 mg
Potassium 117 mg Phosphorus 11 mg

BROWN BAG POPCORN

Ingredients:
Based on 1 serving per recipe.
1/4 cup popcorn kernels
1 teaspoon canola oil
1 brown paper lunch bag
Directions:

1. In a small bowl combine popcorn and oil.
2. Put popcorn in a brown bag, fold to close and staple the top twice.
3. Microwave on high for 3 minutes or until there is 5 seconds between pops

About This Recipe:

Movie night at home is more fun with popcorn. Try this low cost and low sodium recipe. You can add more flavor with no-salt seasoning or Parmesan cheese.

Nutrition Facts (per serving)

Calories 155 Carbohydrates 27 g
Protein 4 g Sodium 0 mg
Potassium 105 mg Phosphorus 96 mg

PITA WEDGES

Ingredients:

Based on 8 servings per recipe.
4 rounds pita bread
butter, margarine, mayonnaise or oil to cover rounds
1/2 cup parmesean cheese, fresh grated
1 teaspoon oregano, dried

Directions:

1. Using a pastry brush or paper towel, spread pita bread with small amount of margarine, butter, or mayonnaise, or spray with a light spray of cooking oil.
2. Sprinkle about 2 tablespoons parmesan cheese and dried herbs on each round.
3. Cut pita bread rounds into 8 sections.
4. Do this by cutting them in half, then half again, then half one more time.

5. Toast in a 450 degree oven for about 3-5 minutes, until cheese melts and chips toast.
6. Serve with low sodium salsa.

Nutrition Facts (per serving)

Calories 104 Carbohydrates 11 g
Protein 3 g Sodium 161 mg
Potassium 30 mg Phosphorus 45 mg

CHICKEN NOOD LE SOUP

Ingredients:

Yield: 8 servings Serving size: ¾ cup
1 pound chicken parts
1 teaspoon red pepper
¼ cup lemon juice
1 teaspoon caraway seed
3 ½ cups water
1 teaspoon oregano
1 tablespoon poultry seasoning
1 teaspoon sugar
1 teaspoon garlic powder
½ cup celery
1 teaspoon onion powder
½ cup green pepper
2 tablespoons vegetable oil
1 cup egg noodles
1 teaspoon black pepper

Directions:

1. Rub chicken parts with lemon juice.
2. In a large pot, combine chicken, water, poultry seasoning, garlic powder, onion powder, vegetable oil, black pepper, red pepper, caraway seed, oregano, and sugar together. Cook 30 minutes or until chicken is tender.
3. Add remaining ingredients and cook for

an additional 15 minutes. Serve hot. Note: Soup may require additional water; if so, add water ½ cup at a time.

Nutrition Facts (per serving)
Calories 110 Carbohydrates 7 g
Protein 3 g Sodium 17 mg
Potassium 101 mg Phosphorus 39 mg

BEEF & VEGETABLE SOUP

Ingredients:
Yield: 8 servings Serving size: ¾ cup
1 pound beef stew
3 ½ cups water
1 cup raw sliced onions
½ cup frozen green peas
1 teaspoon black pepper
½ cup frozen okra
½ teaspoon basil
½ cup frozen carrots, diced
½ teaspoon thyme
½ cup frozen corn
Directions:
1. In a large pot, place beef stew, onions, black pepper, basil, thyme and water. Cook for about 45 minutes.
2. Add all frozen vegetables; simmer on low heat until meat is tender. Serve hot.
Note:
soup may require additional water. Add water ½ cup at a time as necessary.

Nutrition Facts (per serving)
Calories 190 Carbohydrates 7 g
Protein 11 g Sodium 56 mg
Potassium 291 mg Phosphorus 121 mg

SIMPLE CHICKEN BROTH

Ingredients:
Based on tbd servings per recipe.
3 pounds chicken wings or whole chicken
2 onions, halved
1 celery rib, halved
2 carrots, halved
8 peppercorns, whole
2 teaspoons dried thyme
2 bay leaves
Directions:
1. Place all items in a large pot with about 16 cups of cold water.
2. Bring to a boil, then simmer.
3. Skim the froth that comes to the top.
4. Simmer for about 3 hours.
5. Save chicken meat, throw away other solids, and pour broth through a sieve.
6. Add chicken, grains, and vegetables.
7. Simmer for 30 minutes.
8. Can be frozen in portions for up to 3 months

Nutrition Facts (per serving)
Calories 20 Carbohydrates 9 g
Protein 1 g Sodium 67 mg
Potassium 196 mg Phosphorus 55 mg

BEEF BARLEY SOUP

Ingredients:
Based on 10 servings per recipe.
1/2 teaspoon black pepper
2 lbs beef stew meat, diced 1 inch cubes
1/4 cup vegetable oil, divided
1 cup chopped onion
1/2 cup sliced mushrooms

2 carrots, diced
1/2 teaspoon garlic, minced
1/4 teaspoon dried thyme
1 can (14.5 ounces) chicken broth, low sodium
3 cups water
1 frozen package (16 ounces) of vegetables
2 potatoes, soaked and diced
1/2 cup barley

Directions:
1. 1. Season beef with pepper.
2. Add 2 tablespoons oil to stew pot and saute 5 minutes.
3. Add 2 more tablespoons of oil and add onions, carrots and mushrooms.
4. Saute for 5 minutes and stir often.
5. Add garlic and thyme and saute for 3 mins.
6. Add chicken broth and water to pot.
7. Add mixed vegtables, potatoes and barley.
8. Stir and bring to boil.
9. Cover and reduce heat.
10. Simmer 1 to 1 1/2 hours.

Nutrition Facts (per serving)
Calories 270 Carbohydrates 22 g
Protein 23 g Sodium 105 mg
Potassium 678 mg Phosphorus 250 mg

BAKED POTATO SOUP

Ingredients:
Based on 6 (1 1/2 cup each) servings per recipe.
2 large potatoes
1/3 cup flour
4 cups skim milk
1/2 teaspoon pepper

4 ounces, shredded reduce fat monterey jack cheese
1/2 cup fat free sour cream

Directions:
1. Bake potatoes at 400 degrees until fork tender.
2. Let cool.
3. Cut lengthwise and scoop out pulp.
4. Place flour in large sauce pan. Gradually add milk, stirring until blended.
5. Add potato pulp and pepper.
6. Cook over medium heat until thick and bubbly, stirring frequently.
7. Add cheese, stir until cheese melts.
8. Remove from heat and stir in sour cream.

Nutrition Facts (per serving)
Calories 216 Carbohydrates 29 g
Protein 15 g Sodium 272 mg
Potassium 594 mg Phosphorus 326 mg

THAI CHICKEN SOUP

Ingredients:
Based on 6 servings per recipe.
1 pound chicken breast, cut into bite size pieces, or shrimp
4 cups our Simple Chicken Broth recipe or other low sodium broth
1/2 tablespoon fish sauce
1 tablespoon sugar (brown or white)
1 teaspoon chili sauce or chili flakes
1 lemon grass stalk, chopped
1 inch ginger, sliced
1 can lite coconut milk
10 white button mushrooms, quartered
1 red bell pepper, sliced
1/2 yellow onion, sliced

2 tablespoons lime juice
Directions:
1. Spray a large pot with non stick cooking spray and cook chicken or shrimp over medium heat until evenly browned.
2. Add broth, fish sauce, sugar, chili sauce, lemongrass, and ginger.
3. Bring to a boil.
4. Reduce heat to medium-low and let simmer for 10-15 minutes.
5. Add coconut milk, mushrooms, bell pepper, and onion and simmer for another 5 minutes.
6. Stir in lime juice before serving

Nutrition Facts (per serving)
Calories 233 Carbohydrates 9 g
Protein 32 g Sodium 300 mg
Potassium 800 mg Phosphorus 382 mg

DIABETIC COOKBOOK

for Beginners

Diabetic Cookbook with Easy and Healthy Diabetes Meal Prep Recipes
with 28-Day Meal Plan to Manage Type 2 Diabetes Newly Diagnosed

**INCLUDE
28-Day
Meal Plan**

VANCOUVER
PRESS

DIABETIC
COOKBOOK
for Beginners

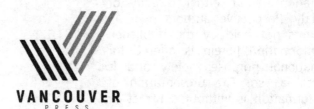

VANCOUVER
PRESS

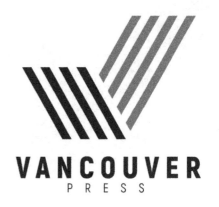

Contents

1. So, What Exactly is Diabetes?...160

2. The 3 Practices That Can Prevent and Reserve Type II
   Diabetes and Manage Type I Diabetes.............................173

3. Healty Lifestyle Habits for Preventing/Beating
   Diabetes (and Other Health Problems)............................176

4. Get Up and Get Moving..191

5. Dieting/Nutrition Tips for Preventing, Managing and
   Reversing Diabetes..206

6. The Overlooked Importance of Staying Hydrated..........221

7. Stress Is a Cause (and Symptom) of Diabetes...............224

8. Assembling a Support Team...227

9. The 5 Words that Turn This Report Into Positive Results...230

10. 28-Day Meal Plan For People with Diabetes................234

11. 50 Mouth-Weatering Diabetic Recipes That Taste
    Like Absolute Heaven...404
   ° *Dibetic Date Dainties*..405
   ° *Sugar - Free Cranberry Relish*................................405
   ° *It Could Be a Snickers Bar*....................................405
   ° *Baked Chiken for One*...405
   ° *Chocolate Chip Cookies*..406
   ° *Brownie Torte*..406
   ° *Frozen Apricot Mousse*..406
   ° *Raspberry Mousse*..406
   ° *Fanciful Freeze*..407

° No-Sugar Custard 407
° Orange Sherbert (For Diabetics) 407
° Diabetic Apple Pie 407
° Strawberry Diabetic Jam 408
° Diabetic Punch 408
° No Bake Diabetic Fruit Cake 408
° Diabetic Raisin Cake 408
° Diabetic Sponge Cake 409
° Mary Tyler Moore's Almond Meringue Cookies (Diabetic) 409
° Diabetic Bread Pudding 409
° Diabetic Peanut Butter Cookies 410
° Diabetic Brownies 410
° Diabetic Jelly 410
° Anne's Diabetic Chocolate Syrup 411
° Diabetic Cinnamon Cookies 411
° Diabetic Easter Fudge 411
° Spiced Tea (Diabetic) 411
° Diabetic Cranberry and Orange Salad 412
° Diabetic Glorified Rice 412
° Diabetic Cream Cheese Salad 412
° Easy Sugar-Free Dessert 413
° Cream Puffs 413
° Sugarless Apple Pie 413
° Smakeroon Cookies 413
° Chocolate Sauce 414
° Dietetic Pasta Salad 414
° Sugar Free Apple Pie 414
° Diabetic Cheese Cake 415
° Diabetic Pumpkin Pie 415
° Diabetic Whipped Cream 415
° Strawberry Pie (No sugar) 415
° Popsicles 416
° Polish Sausage Stew 416
° Krautrunza 416
° German Sauerkraut 416

° Patchlinghs 417
° Walnut Dreams 417
° Mom's Wiener Soup 417
° Iocoa Egg Pancakes 417
° Tuna Supreme 418
° Diabetic Spicy 418
° Pork Chops & Stuffing 418
° Banana Bread 418
° Buttermilk Sherbet 418

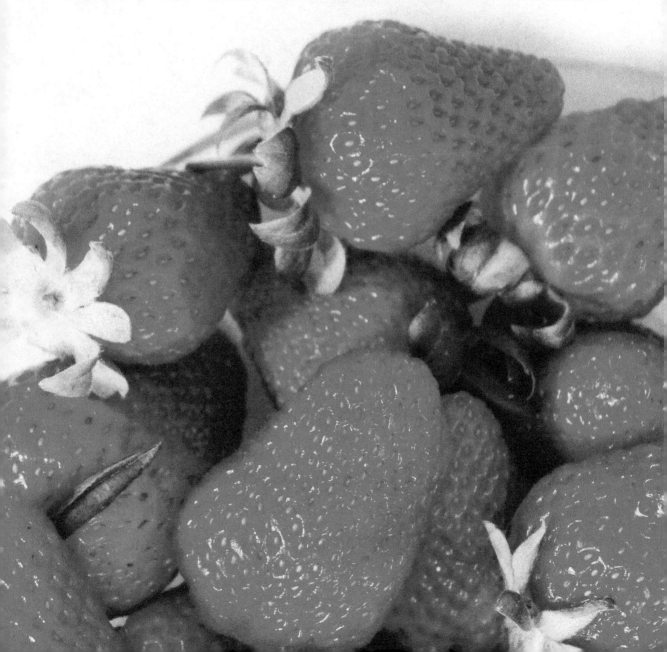

1

So, What Exactly is Diabetes?

Diabetes is a blood sugar problem. The glucose (sugar) in the food you eat stays in your blood rather than going into your cells where it can be used as energy. Different Types of diabetes develop because of different causes. We will talk about what causes diabetes in just a bit. For now, let's see what a respected health authority has to say on the matter. The Centers for Disease Control (CDC) in the US tells us this about diabetes:

"Diabetes is a condition in which the body does not properly process food for use as energy. When you have diabetes, your body either doesn't make enough insulin or can't use its own

it should. This causes sugar to build up in your blood. Diabetes can cause serious health complications including heart disease, blindness, kidney failure, and lower extremity amputations. Diabetes is the seventh leading cause of death in the United States."

DiabetesResearch.org shares these alarming facts and figures about diabetes:

- Diabetes now affects more than 422 million people around the world.

- 70 million Americans have prediabetes and an additional 30 million have diabetes. That means 1 in every 3.6 people in the US is either prediabetic or diabetic.

- 1 in 4 people with diabetes don't even know they have this health condition which can lead to so many other problems.

- In the first 15 years of the 21st century, the number of people living with diabetes has increased by nearly 50%.

To say that diabetes is an epidemic is possibly the greatest understatement of this young century. Type 1 and Type 2 diabetes are the most common forms of this disease, and what we will be addressing in this report. Gestational diabetes affects 2% to 5% of pregnant women, and usually disappears after birth.

How Is Diabetes Diagnosed?

The most commonly used tool to diagnose diabetes is the glycated hemoglobin (A1C) test. Your doctor uses this blood test to discover what your average blood sugar level has been for the past two or three months. Your blood sugar can spike from time to time. Certain foods cause a release of more glucose than others, so after a meal you may experience an elevated blood sugar level. Your blood sugar can also drop below healthy levels every now and then.

Experiencing high blood sugar is not a sign of prediabetes or diabetes if it is infrequent. What the A1C test does is indicate whether or not you have a chronic blood sugar problem. You can ask your doctor at any time to perform an A1C test so you can find out if your blood sugar level is in a healthy range.

If your test shows a level of 5. 7% or lower, this is considered normal and healthy. If you test between 5.7% and 6.4%, this is an indication of prediabetes. A result of 6.5% or higher means that you are diabetic.

Are there alternatives to the A1C Test?

If you have an uncommon form of hemoglobin or if for some reason an A1C test is not available, your doctor will turn to one of the following diabetes testing alternatives.

- **Fasting blood sugar test** – Your doctor will take a blood sample after you have fasted for at least 12 hours. If the result of that test shows less than 100 milligrams per deciliter (mg/dL) of glucose in your blood, congratulations. This is normal. A level of 100 to 125 mg/dL is a sign of prediabetes, and over 126 mg/dL signals diabetes.

- **Random blood sugar test** – Instead of asking you to fast, your doctor may take a random blood sugar test at any time. This may be because of scheduling difficulties, when you are not able to perform a fast before getting a fasting blood sugar test. Regardless of when you may have eaten last, a blood sugar reading of 200 mg/dL or higher will bring a diagnosis of diabetes,

- as long as there are multiple symptoms present.

- **Oral glucose tolerance test** – This test is not very common. Like the fasting blood sugar test, you will be asked to go without eating for a certain period of time. Your doctor will have you drink a sweet, sugary liquid concoction, after which your blood sugar level will be tested several times over the next two hours. A reading of less than 140 mg/dL is normal. If you score between 140 and 199, this is an indication of prediabetes. A reading of over 200 after the two hour testing period suggests that you have diabetes.

Let's get to know a little bit more about diabetes, and then we will share with you tips and best practices proven to prevent diabetes from developing, treat it if you already have diabetes, and in some cases reverse the condition entirely.

What Are the Differences between Type I and Type II Diabetes?

Type I Diabetes

Type I diabetes is more serious than Type II. This was in the past referred to as juvenile diabetes, since it usually forms in kids and teenagers. It is sometimes called insulin-dependent diabetes mellitus (IDDM). However, Type I diabetes can develop at any age.

When you have Type I diabetes, your body's defense system attacks the pancreas. Your immune system for some strange reason identifies the pancreas as an enemy agent. Scientists are not totally sure why this happens. Even though we don't know the cause, we understand the experience.

Type I diabetes causes your immune system to identify the pancreas as a foreigner that doesn't belong. It is viewed as an invader. The job of your immune system is to keep threats out of the body and to repel disease and illness. In its attempt to do its job properly, it improperly begins to attack and destroy the cells of the pancreas.

Your pancreas cells, called islets, have a very important job. Their main task is to identify glucose in your blood. Once that glucose is recognized, the islets begin producing the correct amount of insulin to normalize your blood sugar level. Insulin is required to open up the cells in your body to allow glucose to enter. This glucose is used for energy.

Without insulin, there is no opening of the cells to receive glucose. This is what causes Type I diabetes to let sugar stay in your blood and build up until it is at dangerously high levels.

Additionally, the cells throughout your body are starving from a lack of glucose. If this condition is not treated, the high blood sugar which is the major symptom of Type I diabetes can lead to vision problems, damage to your nerves and kidneys, heart disease and other cardiovascular conditions, lower extremity amputation, and in some cases produce a coma and even death.

Because of this inherent problem inside the body to regulate the glucose/insulin relationship, those with Type I diabetes need to take insulin injections. The insulin level in the human body can be influenced by diet, physical activity level, stress, emotions and overall fitness. Since these factors can change frequently, even hourly in some cases, a person's glucose level needs to be closely monitored throughout the day.

This next statistic is very important!

- **Type I diabetes accounts for just 5% to 10% of all diagnosed cases of diabetes.**

Type II Diabetes

Type II diabetes (non-insulin-dependent diabetes mellitus or NIDDM) accounts for 90% to 95% of all diabetes cases.

That actually is a good statistic, because in nearly every case, Type II diabetes can be prevented.It can be avoided by making smart lifestyle choices, eating right and exercising.
In many cases, Type II diabetes can also be reversed using these same practices, which is exactly what we are going to teach you in this report.

Type II diabetes used to be referred to as adult onset diabetes because it generally happens in adults. Nearly 4 out of every 10 Type II sufferers need insulin injections. Physical inactivity, obesity, a poor diet, older age and a family history of diabetes are just a few of the risk factors someone may experience that raise the risk of developing Type II diabetes.

Unlike Type I diabetes, there usually is a not a problem with insulin production or reception. This is wonderful news, because it means as long as you take action on the information in this report, you can prevent diabetes from happening. If it does develop, you can reverse the condition and enjoy health and wellness once again.

Common Diabetes Symptoms

We discussed how diabetes keeps your body from using energy properly. It stores sugar (glucose, your body's favorite energy source) in your blood rather than letting it get to your cells, where it is needed. Because of this one of the most common diabetes symptoms is chronic fatigue.

You feel like you never have any energy. Even after pounding coffee and getting lots of rest, you feel extremely fatigued after performing very little or no physical activity. Here are a few of the other more common diabetes symptoms.

- Overweight and obesity
- You have to urinate often
- You are constantly very thirsty, and this is a thirst which is stronger than normal
- You feel hungry even though you are eating, or immediately after eating
- Blurred vision, changes in vision ability
- When you get a bruise or a cut, it is very slow to heal

- You become sick or infected more than usual
- With Type II diabetes, a tingling or numbness in the hands and feet is a sign of diabetes or prediabetes
- With Type I diabetes, you may experience unexplained weight loss, even if you attempt to eat more and more to keep this from happening
- With Type I diabetes, vomiting, nausea and stomach pains may occur at the onset of the condition

If you display one or two of these symptoms from time to time, there may not be a serious issue. When you experience 2 or more of these classic diabetes symptoms regularly, it is highly recommended that you let your doctor know. Early diagnosis and treatment produces the best results with any Type of diabetes.

Who Gets Diabetes?

In 5 or 10 out of every 100 diabetes cases, diabetes occurs because of a developmental problem in the human body. This is Type I diabetes. In the other 90 or 95 cases out of every 100, behaviors and lifestyle choices lead to the formation of diabetes.

- As mentioned above, if there is a history of diabetes in your family, your risk is higher than normal. American Indians and African-Americans have a much higher diabetes risk factor than other races. If a woman has gestational diabetes (diabetes during pregnancy) she is at an increased risk for developing Type II diabetes later on. Pacific Islanders have a higher probability of developing diabetes than many other cultural groups.

Less common forms of diabetes develop because of a reaction to drugs, malnutrition, infections or other illnesses, and even after surgery. These are extremely rare, making up only 1% or 2% of all diabetes cases.

In as many as 9 out of 10 cases or more, the person who develops diabetes does so because of poor lifestyle choices, a poor diet and poor physical fitness practices. This means you can not only prevent it, but also reverse the condition once you are diagnosed.

The information contained here can help those suffering from Type I diabetes better manage their condition, so they enjoy the best possible health and wellness. For preventing or reversing Type II diabetes, this same information is extremely successful and has been for men and women, young and old, and can produce results quickly.

Can I Stop Prediabetes so It Doesn't BecomeType II Diabetes?

What is prediabetes? This is a situation where blood glucose levels are slightly elevated above what would be considered normal. Prediabetes can come and go, and is a predictor of an eventual development of Type II diabetes if certain steps are not taken. Prediabetes (and diabetes, for that matter) can only be uncovered during a checkup with your doctor.

Look at the list of diabetes symptoms we discussed earlier. An infrequent appearance of some of those symptoms could be an indicator of prediabetes.

Fortunately, the prediabetic person can employ a 3-pronged treatment plan that cannot only keep Type II diabetes from developing, but can also dramatically lower the risk of developing cancer, heart disease, obesity, diabetes and several other major health problems.

Let's take a look at the three simple but extremely important practices for successfully preventing and treating diabetes.

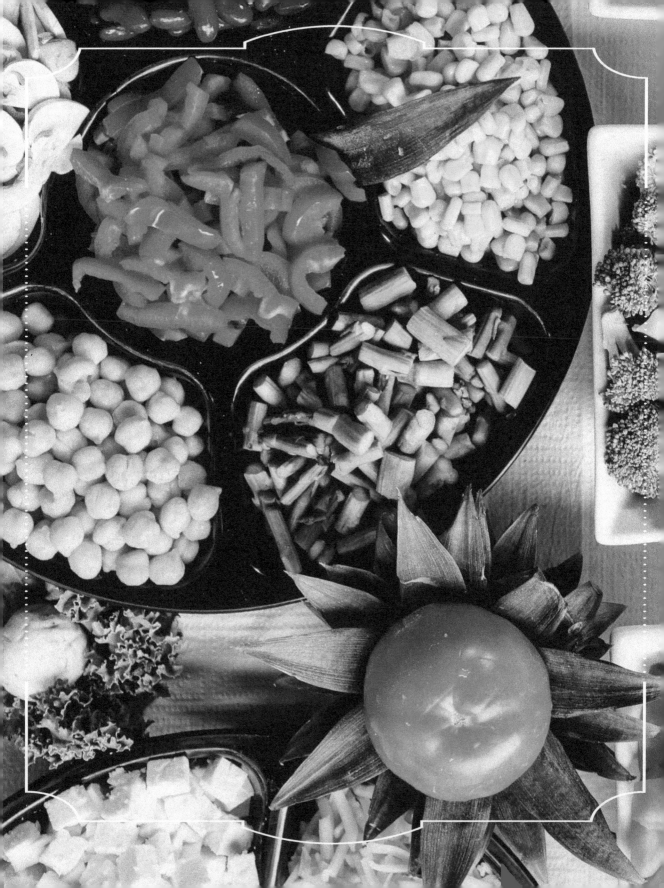

2

The 3 Practices That Can Prevent and Reverse Type II Diabetes and Manage Type I Diabetes

Research announced on MedicalNewsToday.com and elsewhere in late 2018 is very promising regarding the reversal of Type I diabetes. Many researchers and doctors are on the verge of generating insulin-making cells that might possibly reverse the insulin sensitivity and creation process that happens with Type I diabetes.

At this point in time though, there is no total cure forType I diabetes.

However, there are 3 areas in your life where you can take action to treat Type I diabetes, and either prevent or reverse Type II diabetes. These three factors which dictate much of your physical and mental health and well-being are:

- Lifestyle Behaviors
- How Active You Are
- What You Eat and Drink

Over the next 3 sections of your report, we will dig deeply into each of these influential health and wellness factors. They are so important for treating and preventing diabetes, obesity, heart disease, brain-based health problems, cancer and a number of other serious diseases and illnesses. Let's discuss some healthy lifestyle changes you can make to give you the upper hand in your fight against diabetes.

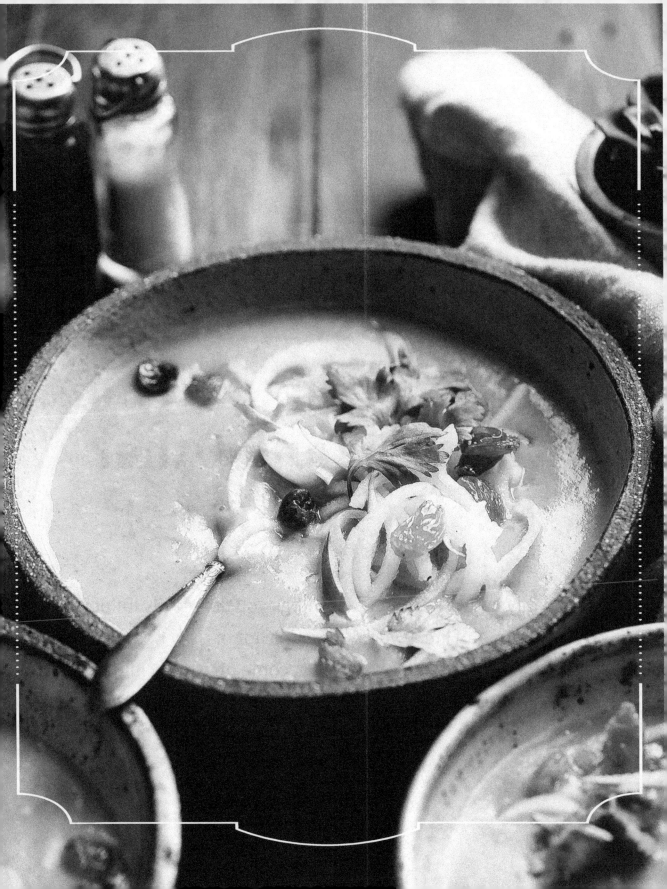

3

Healthy Lifestyle Habits for Preventing/Beating Diabetes (and Other Health Problems)

You probably understand that the things you do heavily influence what you get out of life. If you engage in a lot of risky behavior, you are more likely than most people to become physically injured, arrested or receive some negative consequences for your actions.

The opposite is also true. If you avoid danger and risks, you stand a better chance than average of the living a longer life. In other words the way in which you live and the decisions you make are largely responsible for the quality of life you enjoy.

Are you good at saving money?

This may not seem to be applicable for a guide on how to prevent and treat diabetes. However, your money management skills can be used as an example to show how the decisions you make and the activities you engage in can deliver either a positive or negative end result.

If you spend money wisely and always save some of your income, you probably will be able to retire before someone who makes the same amount of money but doesn't have those skills. You might not exercise the smartest money management practices. You figure that you might as well spend the money while you have it, and you never put away anything for a rainy day.

In the second example, you may never get to retire. You may have to work until the day you die to pay bills and keep a roof over your head. You also won't have any money tucked away for a rainy day or an emergency.

In both of those examples about handling your finances, you see how decisions lead to a very predictable end result.

This is what happens in the case of Type II diabetes.

If you eat mostly highly processed food, you are sedentary and not very active, you don't have healthy sleep habits and you drink alcohol in excess, those lifestyle behaviors virtually guarantee you are going to encounter prediabetes or Type II diabetes eventually.

Even the most amazing immune system and the healthiest organs and internal processes can't battle an unhealthy diet, poor exercise habits and negative lifestyle activities forever.

While your decisions concerning diet and exercise are far and away the most important in determining whether or not you will develop diabetes, there are other lifestyle choices you make which can improve or lower your health and well-being in a number of ways. Here are a few recommendations that can help you treat, beat and reverse diabetes, while simultaneously making you healthier overall.

Socialize

People have a natural tendency to herd. It's true. People are more likely to seek out others than to live a life of solitude. This behavior of most people goes back to the earliest humans. In the cave dwelling period of human development, the daily struggle to survive was very real.

You and I fortunately don't have to contend with the myriad of problems our Paleo ancestors faced. For them, each day was a true test of survival.The many threats to humans meant that people had a better chance of surviving if they formed a group. A group of several human beings could hunt, gather and defend themselves against other humans better than if those early humans were attempting to survive individually. This is what created the world's first societies.

Fast-forward to modern times and people still have an inborn desire to socialize.

Several studies have shown that human touch causes the release of hormones that make us feel happy. This happens if that touch is a handshake or a hug, a kiss on the cheek or simply making physical contact with someone you are comfortable around in some other way. "Feel-good" hormones and chemicals are released, and "feel-bad" chemicals are depleted. This is one of the very many real benefits of socialization for beating or treating diabetes.

Stress is a major cause and symptom of diabetes. Socializing leads to fewer feelings of stress and anxiety, and more feelings of happiness and belonging.

Start spending more time with your loved ones. Call your friends and chat with them regularly. Join a local civic group. Get "out an about" and mix and mingle. Socializing is a lifestyle habit that can help you cut down on the stress that can aggravate diabetes, and people who are social also enjoy a reduced risk of developing a long list of other mental and physical diseases and illnesses.

Get Regular Checkups

So many health problems are preventable. Negative health conditions such as Type II diabetes, obesity and the problems that accompany it, heart disease and liver disease are preventable for the most part. Sure, there are always going to be factors that cause a health problem to develop that you have no control over.

You may have to deal with some issue because of your genetic history and makeup. You might have a bad reaction to some type of medication or for some other reason experience a serious health problem.

In many cases though, all you have to do is talk with your doctor regularly to see what is going on inside your body. How do you know if you have some condition you have to address if you are not regularly tested for that and other health issues? This means that one lifestyle activity you should definitely adopt if you want to conquer diabetes is to get regular checkups.

Get your blood sugar checked regularly. Type I diabetics do this several times a day. People with Type II diabetes don't consider doing it too frequently because they don't have to inject themselves with insulin, in most cases.

You also want to get your heart health, respiratory system, blood pressure and other important health metrics checked. Monitor them regularly, at least every 6 months. If you have diabetes in your family tree, you should definitely be getting checked up as soon as possible, and then again every 4 to 6 months to develop a plan of action that will give you the most positive end result.

If you have never been diagnosed with diabetes and are experiencing any of the diabetes symptoms we mentioned earlier, like unexplained weight loss, obesity, frequent thirst, extreme fatigue or you have to urinate often, call your doctor and schedule a checkup.

If you are diabetic, you should definitely be seeing your doctor regularly so you can understand what kind of progress you are making in treating this condition.You cannot ignore this situation in the hopes that it will go away. If you don't know if you are diabetic, get a checkup. If you are diabetic, your doctor should have already given you a regular checkup schedule to follow. Either way, whether you are battling Type I diabetes or Type II diabetes, regular checkups are a smart lifestyle practice.

Stop Smoking Tobacco

Smoking isn't good for anyone. It is especially risky for diabetics. Nicotine is one of the many chemicals in cigarettes and e-cigarettes, hookahs and other tobacco products that makes diabetes worse. Aside from being extremely addictive, nicotine (even in second-hand smoke) has been linked to heart disease, pancreatic, esophageal and oral cancer, kidney disease, stroke and heart disease.

One of the negative effects of nicotine on the heart has to do with your blood vessels.

This addictive chemical narrows blood vessels. It makes them harder and more dense. This means your blood doesn't flow as naturally as it should. Since diabetes makes you more likely to develop some type of heart disease, the fact that nicotine makes it even harder for your heart to do its job means smoking unnecessarily raises your risk of suffering a heart attack or stroke.

Looking at the big picture, not just in relation to diabetes, smoking has been provenas a cause of the following health concerns:

- A host of cancers
- Diabetes
- Erectile dysfunction
- Heart disease
- Pregnancy problems

- Loss of vision
- Tuberculosis
- Rheumatoid arthritis
- A weak immune system
- Prematurely aged skin and hair
- Sleep problems
- Weakened bones, less bone density
- Hearing loss
- Poor circulation
- Psoriasis
- Crohn's disease
- Acid reflux
- Premature or sudden death

Is your smoking habit worth it? Look at this partial list of the serious health problems caused by smoking. Are your cigarettes worth experiencing these issues? Did you know smokers live 10 years less than non-smokers, on average? The final years of a smoker's life are painful and full of doctors, numerous ailments and health problems.

Smokers run up $289 million in healthcare costs annually ... in the US alone.

Exposure to secondhand smoke kills hundreds of thousands of people around the world every year. Since it hurts your immune system, you are more likely to get sick from any illness or disease. The average smoker spends a little less than $2,000 on his habit annually, cigarette smoke smells terrible and permeates your clothes and furniture, and smokers are more prone to overeat than non-smokers.

If you are trying to prevent diabetes, treat it or hopefully reverse it, stop smoking. The payoff is a healthier body inside and out ... and a fatter checkbook.

Additionally, every other person who smokes will die from a smoking-related illness, according to the World Health Organization (WHO). That's 1 in every 2 smokers.

That last stat should scare you right out of smoking. Hey, it is tough to stop smoking. There is no doubt about it. It is easier to end your relationship with tobacco when you keep in mind how many ways your health benefits when you do.

Drink Only Moderate Levels of Alcohol

The American Diabetes Association says women who drink alcohol should have no more than one drink a day. They recommend that men should have no more than two. Chronic drinking can lead to short and long-term memory loss, neurological disorders and diseases, unhealthy weight gain, liver disease, high blood pressure and a number of cancers. There are many good reasons for drinking alcohol responsibly, whether you are diabetic or not.

Give Yourself the Gift of Healthy Sleep Habits

When you are fully rested on a regular basis, your mind is sharp and you don't need to turn to unhealthy energy drinks, caffeine and sugar to stay awake and alert. Poor sleep habits have been linked to overweight and obesity, causes and symptoms of diabetes. Aside from boosting your natural energy level, getting plenty of rest boosts your heart health.

We mentioned earlier how diabetics are more prone to developing heart disease than people who are not diabetic. Not regularly getting 7 to 8 hours of restful sleep damages your heart, which means the combination of diabetes and poor sleep habits makes you much more likely to suffer a heart attack, stroke or some other cardiovascular event.

Did you know that at least 7 hours of sleep is required night in and night out for you to enjoy a healthy blood pressure level?

It's true. Your body needs to repair and rest often. When you're asleep, there are a number of bodily processes which naturally occur to get you ready for the following day.

One of these processes is a lowering of your blood pressure. If you do not sleep long enough, your body does not lower your blood pressure properly. This means when you awaken in the morning and you haven't slept enough and let your body recuperate properly, you can wake up to high blood pressure.

If your heart has to work too hard due to elevated blood pressure levels, this raises your risk of developing diabetes. High blood pressure can also exacerbate diabetes if it has already developed. Keeping your heart healthy is important for preventing and treating diabetes.

By the way, several studies have shown that poor sleep patterns leads to less ambition. Your brain is just not rested enough to give you the mental energy that is required for you to exercise. You don't feel like being physically active, and this can lead to overweight and obesity, diabetes, a heart attack, and several other health problems.

Some Simple Tips for Better Sleep

- Sticking to a regular sleep schedule is one of the easiest ways to program your body and mind for a healthy night's rest. Go to bed and arise from sleep at the same time each night and each morning if at all possible.

- Experience natural light throughout the day. This means getting out in nature and letting the sunshine down upon you.

- Exercise regularly. (More on this health booster and diabetes destroyer in the next chapter.) It has been proven that if you exercise in the morning it is easier to fall asleep at night. However, exercising any time during the day is better than no exercise at all if you can't get your workout done in the morning.

- Remove electronics from your bedroom.

- Keep your sleeping environment dark and quiet.

- Cooler temperatures promote sleep better than warmer temperatures.
- Don't eat or drink within 3 or more hours of bedtime. Alcohol and foods high in sugar can keep you awake. Drinking any beverage before bedtime can wreck your sleep entirely if you have to get up in the middle of the night to relieve yourself.

Avoid computer screens, your smartphone display and your television within a few hours of bedtime. If you must use your computer or phone, employ a bluelight filter application. Artificial light at nighttime can make it difficult for you to go to sleep.

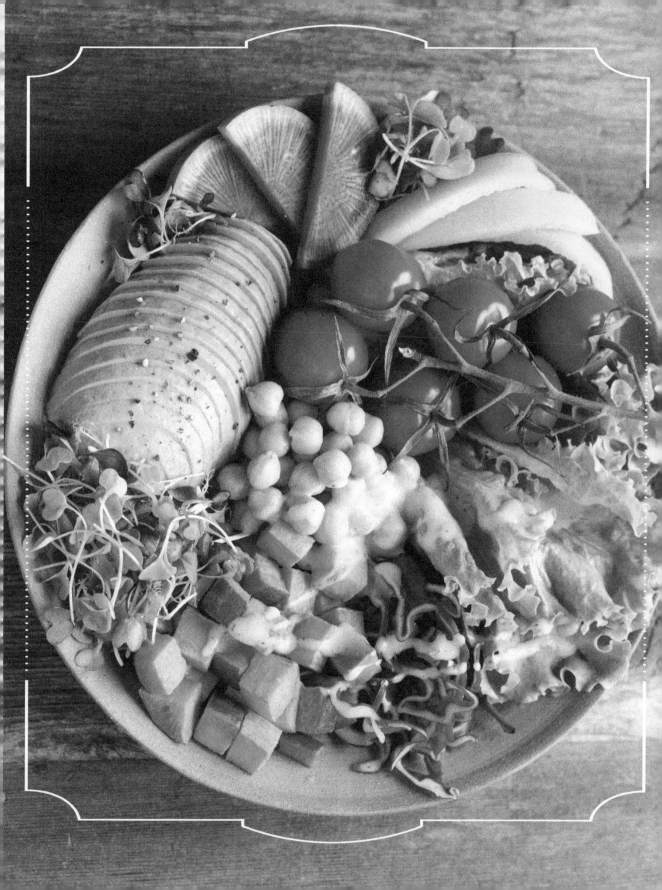

4

Get Up and Get Moving

The human body was not made for sitting.

It was made to be moving most of the time. Unfortunately, many lifestyles and occupations these days lead to hour after hour of sitting. Each morning when you arise from your bed, you prepare for work and end up sitting in your vehicle. You then get out of your car for the short walk to your office or some other work location … and you take a seat.

At the end of the day you sit back down in your car, head home, sit in your favorite seat or on the cozy couch and watch television.

This typical routine for many people has led to the fact that *most Americans sit for an astonishing 13 hours each day.*

Your body was not made for this. It is okay to sit from time to time in order to rest. If you stood up every minute that you weren't asleep, that would not be very healthy. You need to sit down every now and then. The problem is not only sitting vs. standing, but actually what you are doing when you're standing. Humans enjoy their best health and wellness when they are physically active much of the time.

Doctors who are diabetes specialists, fitness gurus and other health professionals recognize regular physical activity as one of the keys to beating diabetes. Exercise regularly and you can improve your health from head to toe. This section of your report covers proven ways to become more physically active so you get the upper hand on diabetes.

How Your Chair Is Killing You

You know how deadly smoking can be. Did you know that there is something you do for hours every day that might just be more dangerous than smoking? "Sitting is the new smoking." That is a statement made by Dr. James Levine, who has dedicated his life to getting the message out about the negative health consequences of sitting for too long.

"Sitting is more dangerous than smoking, kills more people than HIV and is more treacherous than parachuting. We are sitting ourselves to death."

That is a quote from Levine, author of the book "Get up! Why Your Chair Is Killing You and What You Can Do about It."

Dr. Levine works with the globally respected Mayo Clinic in the United States. He has performed significant research over more than 25 years that shows how deadly chronic sitting can be. Again, as we mentioned earlier, it's not necessarily the sitting that is the problem. It is the fact that you are not moving while you are sitting.

Then there are also the number of health conditions that are caused by poor circulation. The longer you sit, the more pressure you are putting on the veins and arteries in your leg. This does not allow for proper circulation of your blood throughout your body. It is also difficult to allow your respiratory system to work properly when seated. When you are standing and moving, you naturally promote healthy cardiovascular, circulatory and respiratory functions.

This is not the case when you're sitting.

Levine found that, *"Those individuals who are lean are up and walking about 2.25 hours more (each day)than those individuals who are obese."* Being overweight and obese are considered gateway health conditions which can lead to diabetes, heart disease and cancer, among other serious health problems. What can you do to combat the fact that your chair may be trying to end your life prematurely?

Get up and get moving after sitting for 20 or 30 minutes.

Perform your daily activities standing and moving whenever you can, as opposed to sitting. Take the stairs at work instead of the elevator. If you leave work or your home for lunch during the day, take a walk instead of driving the car. Ride a bike to and from work if you can. Stand up and fold the laundry, stand when you do the dishes or prepare dinner, or while you are watching your favorite reality show.

Levine's research shows that consciously cutting back on how much you sit each day by just a couple of hours can lead to a 15% to 25% reduced risk of developing diabetes and other significant health problems.

For those that have diabetes, trading physical activity and movement for sitting can help manage symptoms, and in some cases can even begin a reversal of Type II diabetes.

How Much Exercise Promotes Health and Wellness? (It's less than you might think)

At this point, you may be wondering how often you need to be up and moving. What type of physical activity is the best for treating and preventing diabetes? Do you need to spend a lot of money on an expensive gym membership? Maybe you should purchase thousands of dollars of fitness equipment and build a home gymnasium?

Once you make a commitment to being more active regularly in order to manage or prevent diabetes, exactly how many hours a week does that commitment look like?

You may be surprised at the answer to that last question.

The Mayo Clinic, the World Health Organization (WHO) and Britain's National Health Services agree that you only need to engage in 150 minutes of moderately intense exercise each week for maximum health benefits.

That is a total of just 2.5 hours of exercise over 7 days, or just over 20 minutes per day! Isn't that great news?

Research shows it doesn't matter how you break up that activity, either. You can go 30 minutes at a time 5 days per week or exercise for 15 minute sessions 10 times a week. You just need to get to that magic number of 150 weekly minutes to realize significant health benefits.

What was also revealed was that if the activity you are performing is very intense, you need just 75 weekly minutes to get the same benefits.

What is moderately intense physical activity as opposed to intense exercise?

A brisk walk or bike ride is moderate exercise. Running or doing aerobics is intense. Mowing your yard is moderately intense for most people, while attempting to achieve a new personal best in the weight room would be intense and vigorous.

Exercise helps regulate blood sugar levels, it makes you heart and mind stronger and more capable, and regular exercise lowers the odds that you will contract any disease or illness. We are not talking about running marathons, cycling up a mountainside or lifting two times your body weight in the gym either.

Just do something that gets your heart pumping, your body moving, and you huffing and puffing. Here is a simple way to ensure you are engaging in moderately intense exercise ... use the Talk Test.

Take the "Exercise Talk Test" to Reveal How Intense Your Exercise Is

How can you tell if your movements qualify as moderately intense? Take the exercise Talk Test.

The exercise talk test is used to measure the intensity of your physical activity. The harder your heart is beating, your lungs are pumping and your body is moving, the harder it is to carry on a normal conversation. By monitoring how easy or hard it is for you to talk while exercising, you can measure your physical intensity level.

If you can talk with someone while exercising, this is a moderately intense workout. If your speech has to be interrupted by deep breaths and it is impossible to carry on a conversation without interruptions and rest, you are enjoying a vigorous, intense level of exertion.

Don't worry. You don't need to invite someone to work out or exercise with you. It can be fun to get your physical activity requirements while enjoying the company of a friend, but this is not necessary. You can simply talk out loud to yourself to discover what level of intensity you are benefiting from. And by the way, if you hate the idea of exercise, here is some good news.

Any Physical Activity Can Be Exercise

Don't think of exercise as a four letter word. The instant the word exercise is mentioned, a lot of people have negative thoughts. They think this means they're going to have to join an expensive gym or buy a lot of exercise equipment. While traditional exercises, health clubs and gymnasiums can help you treat and beat diabetes, they are by no means necessary for you to get the movement you need.

Any moderately intense physical activity qualifies as exercise.

This means that gardening can be exercise. Playing with your kids or grandkids is a wonderful form of exercise that also delivers emotional benefits. Taking a brisk walk while you are having a conversation with a dear friend means you are getting the right kind of physical activity that can benefit your body and your mind. Dancing, taking a hike and enjoying a bike ride are all forms of exercise.

Strength Training for Preventing, Treating and Beating Diabetes

If you are unhealthy in any way, your risk of developing diabetes or some other significant health problem arises. The healthier you make yourself, in mind and body, the less likely you are to experience diabetes. Doctors and other health professionals experienced with diabetes will tell you that strength training can make your experience with this condition much easier to handle.

There are many reasons why weightlifting, bodyweight exercises and other forms of strength training are good for preventing and treating diabetes. Let's take a look at some of the benefits of strength training if you are diabetic, or you are hoping to prevent prediabetes and diabetes.

- **Less Abdominal Fat** – Harvard researchers reported in 2014 that they had tracked the physical activities of more than 10,000 men. They followed the physical fitness regimen of these men for 12 years. The study revealed that strength training is better than cardiovascular and aerobic exercises for burning abdominal fat. This is important because the more abdominal fat you have, the more pressure that is put on your organs, and the greater your chance of developing diabetes.

- **Increased Heart Health** – Strength training is awesome as a form of exercise because you benefit greatly after a short period of time. Rather than running on your treadmill for an hour, you can strength train in just a few minutes. This means that the better heart health which is delivered by frequent exercise is your companion after just a short period of time when you strength train.

- **Healthy Blood Sugar Levels** – Strength training (sometimes referred to as resistance training) is often recommended for people with Type II diabetes. A study was published in the health journal BioMed Research International in 2013 which showed that strength training maximizes the human body's ability to absorb and use glucose. This a lowers the amount of sugar in your blood, and can help you maintain healthy blood sugar levels.

When you have strong muscles, you have less of a chance of being injured, and improved mobility and flexibility. Strength training makes your bones stronger, and a 2015 study reported in The Lancet revealed that strength training can give you a longer lifespan.

Those are excellent reasons for the nondiabetic or diabetic person to add a strength training regimen to his or her fitness routine. Additionally, strength training has been linked to a reduced risk of developing cancer and improved mental health.

4 Simple (but Health-Boosting) Bodyweight Training Exercises

We just mentioned how important strength training can be for preventing and treating diabetes. Unfortunately, a lot of people don't like to lift heavy weights. You may not want to join a gym because the big, muscled bodies around you can be intimidating, gym memberships can be expensive, and you may have to travel a good distance to and from a health club or gym to lift weights.

Don't worry, there is good news if you want to benefit from the many health rewards of strength training.

Bodyweight exercises replace weights with your body. The weight of your body is your fitness equipment. By combining resistance, gravity and your physical body, you can strength train without fitness equipment or machines. Here are a few simple bodyweight exercises you can do just about anywhere.

- **The Squat** –You squat all the time. You lower your body by bending your knees and spreading your feet, keeping the upper part of your body centered over your legs. You do this to pick things up off the floor, to tie your shoes and perform other common daily activities. The squat works multiple muscle groups and is the perfect bodyweight training exercise for veteran strength trainers and beginners alike.

- **The Plank** –This requires you to get down on the ground. Lie down facing the floor and support yourself on your forearms, the front of your legs, your stomach and chest, and the tips of your toes. Slowly raise your body so your back is straight and stiff, and you are only supported by your toes and your forearms. Hold for 15 seconds and return to the starting position.

- **The Lunge** –This is a great workout for your lower body that also increases balance and core stability. Stand with your feet just about shoulder-width apart. Keeping your back straight and your head facing forward, step far enough forward with one leg so that the trailing leg drops your knee almost to the ground. Hold this position for a few seconds, return to the starting position, and then perform with your other leg.

- **The Push-Up** – Yes, the humble push-up is a great exercise to build muscle strength and mass. Lie face down on the ground, placing your hands palm down at your sides partially under your upper arms. Keeping your legs and back stiff and straight, push off the ground and elevate your body. Return to the starting position.

Doing these 4 simple bodyweight exercises in succession is a great beginners strength training workout. If you can get to the point where you can do 10 to 15 of each of these resistance movements per session for 3 sessions in a row, you are going to like the way you look and feel thanks to the many benefits of strength training.

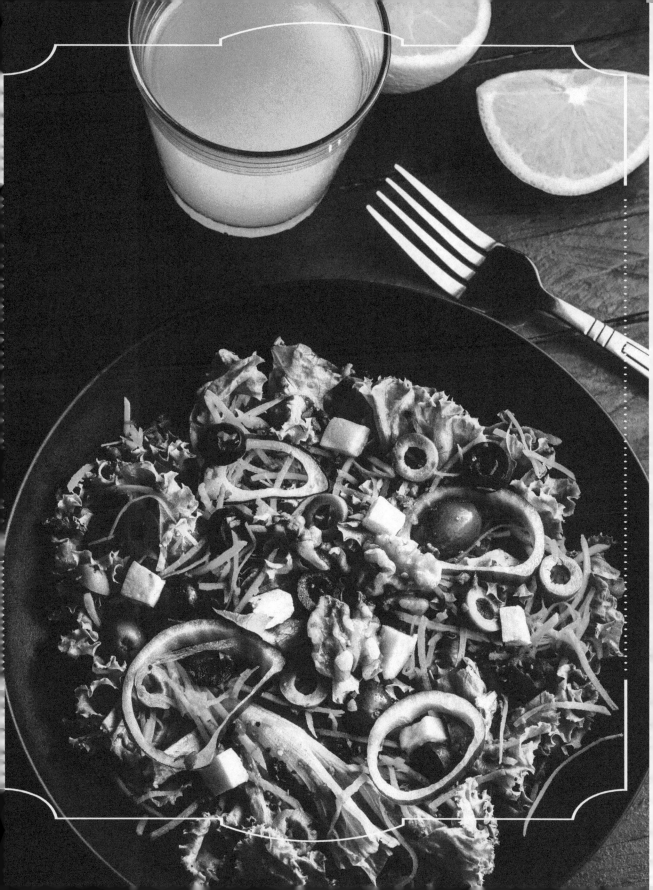

5

Dieting/Nutrition Tips for Preventing, Managing and Reversing Diabetes

If you take only one thing away from this health-boosting report on diabetes, it should be this:

Your diet is the single most important influencer when it comes to your health.

Read that again … then again. If all you do after reading this report is adopt a super-healthy diet, you will enjoy exceptionally better health and wellness, in mind and body.

Fitness gurus, personal trainers and nutritionists will all tell you that the foods and beverages you put into your body have the biggest impact on your health. Exercise is definitely a must if you're going to be as healthy as you can be. You need to sleep regularly, avoid stress and stay hydrated to improve your health as well.

However, your diet is the most powerful single factor for determining how healthy you will be.

This cannot be overstated.

Many health experts agree **that as much as 60% to 75% of your overall fitness, mentally and physically, is determined by what you eat.** Think about it. How many times have you heard about a particular diet for delivering a very specific health result? This is because whatever you decide to give your body as fuel has a direct result on how healthy your mind and body can be.

As far as preventing diabetes is concerned, eating right is an easy way to reach your goal. Remember, as many as 90 to 95 out of every 100 cases of diabetes is Type II.

This Type of diabetes is nearly always preventable … and reversible.

We know that the single biggest cause of Type II diabetes is a poor diet. Eat the wrong kinds of foods and you damage your heart health, you become overweight or obese, you develop diabetes or you suffer from a long list of other health problems.

When that happens, the damage you have done to your body and your mind make you more likely to develop diabetes. An unhealthy body is more prone to becoming diabetic than a healthy body. If it sounds like we are repeating over and over how important a diet is for you to live a healthy, happy and fulfilling life, we are intentionally doing so. What you choose to put into your body will create the health and life you experience.

Let's look at a few different ways you can identify what foods you should be eating (and avoiding) as a diabetic, or if you are trying to keep from developing diabetes.

The Important Difference between Good and Bad Carbohydrates

You are probably familiar with people telling you that one type of food is good and another kind is bad. This is the case with carbohydrates. Many diets will say that simple carbohydrates are bad for you and complex carbohydrates are good for you. In a very basic argument, this is a true statement. The nutrition provided by complex carbohydrates is always going to be higher in value and quantity than what you get out of simple carbohydrates.

However, to say that one carbohydrate is bad and another is good is not really correct.

Food is not bad or good. Some food is better than other choices that you may make at mealtime. You can eat less than healthy food every now and then if you don't overdo it in most cases. Instead of saying good and bad carbohydrates, let's talk about complex (good) carbs and their simple (bad) brethren.

How to Spot Simple and Complex Carbohydrates

Carbohydrates are sugars. Diabetes is a sugar problem. Too much sugar stays in the blood instead of going to the cells where it can be used for energy. Since carbohydrates are sugars and diabetes is a sugar problem, this means that knowing how to identify complex and simple carbohydrates could be the most important nutritional talent you can develop for preventing, treating and possibly reversing diabetes.

- **Simple Carbs** – Simple carbohydrates are also called simple sugars. The word "simple" refers to how the carbohydrate is constructed. It's not very complex. This means it is quickly and easily broken down in the human body. Simple carbohydrates are found in some fruits and vegetables, and also in milk. They are additionally found in abundant levels in highly processed foods. Simple sugars are processed so rapidly that they are often stored in fat cells before they go through the total digestive process. These simply constructed carbohydrates provide no nutrition and only act as energy sources. Eat too many simple carbs on a regular basis and you dramatically raise your risk of developing diabetes. If a person is diabetic, it is imperative that simple carbohydrates are restricted or avoided entirely.

- **Complex Carbs** – Complex carbs are, well … complex. They are constructed in such a detailed way that they are difficult for your body to break down. This means they don't pass into your bloodstream nearly as quickly as simple carbs. Complex carbs are also called starches. Most complex carbohydrates deliver a lot of health and nutrition, and can be found in whole grain foods and starchy vegetables. Because complex carbohydrates take a longer time to digest than simple sugars, there is plenty of time for your body to absorb the nutrition, minerals, vitamins and nutrients they provide. A healthy diet will always include many more foods with complex carbohydrates than simple carbs.

Speaking of carbohydrates, let's take a look at what is undeniably the most dangerous and potentially deadly simple carbohydrate of all.

Sugar – The Sweetest Killer

Did you know that sugar is present in 60% of all food found in American grocery stores? It's true. A group of researchers at the University of North Carolina in 2016 found that 6 out of every 10 items of food in grocery stores throughout America contain added sugar. In many cases, the amount of sugar added is much too high to be healthy, and in many cases sugar was added to foods that you wouldn't think had sugar as an ingredient.

You expect sugar in cookies, soft drinks and energy drinks, but did you know ketchup contains sugar? There is sugar in pasta sauce, salad dressing and even bread. By the way, in the study we just mentioned, the researchers wanted to find out how many processed food items contained added sugar. They looked at their data and removed fresh produce like fruits and vegetables, as well as any other food that was not processed at all, or minimally processed.

They found high levels of sugar added to 68% of highly processed food.

Incidentally, sugar is a simple carbohydrate. When you eat a fruit that has a natural sugar in it, you receive dietary fiber, minerals, nutrients, vitamins and other wonderfully healthy ingredients. The sugar has a minimal impact because it is accompanied by an abundance of nutrition.

Not only that, but the presence of sugar in processed foods and beverages is much higher in almost every instance than it is when found in naturally healthy foods.

Multiple health authorities around the world recommend that women should consume no more than 6 teaspoons of sugar every day. Men should not get more than 9 teaspoons per day.

This includes sugars found in fruits, natural honey and other foods that come from nature. It also includes added sugars that are hidden in highly processed foods, as well as the refined sugar you intentionally add to recipes and your coffee.

Unfortunately, there are sickeningly high and unhealthy levels of sugar in a lot of common food and drink items.

- 12 ounce Coke or similar soft drink – 8 to 9 teaspoons
- 12 ounce Red Bull and other energy drinks – 7 to 10 teaspoons
- 1 tablespoon of catchup – 1 teaspoon
- 6 ounces of yogurt – up to 7 teaspoons
- Single serving of some salad dressings – 4 to 5 teaspoons

There is added sugar in whole-wheat bread, breading and coating mixes, peanut butter and tomato sauce, baked beans and crackers. You can find added sugar in pancake mix, crackers and baked goods. Food manufacturers use sugar because it is a powerfully addictive chemical that is cheap and long-lasting. Because it is so addictive, they add it to just about everything they make.

When you limit the amount of sugar you put into your body, you automatically lower the amount of sugar that goes into your bloodstream. If you eliminated refined sugar from your diet entirely, you would not be missing out on any nutrition. You would limit the chances that you develop diabetes, obesity, heart disease, cancer and many other health problems linked to sugar.

Not All Fats Are Bad ... Really!

In the 1960s and 1970s, sugar manufacturers told us eating fat was bad. They totally avoided mentioning the fact that your body must have certain fats for you to survive. Essential fatty acids are one example of fats that you need to be healthy.

What "Big Sugar"did was spend tons of money saying that fat was bad for you, and sugar was part of a healthy diet. In the decades since, several reports have been brought to light that show how food manufacturers and sugar producers knowingly lied about the devastatingly bad effect sugar has on human health and well-being. In some cases, scientists were paid to misreport test results and research, all in pursuit of the almighty dollar.

We know now that there are healthy fats and unhealthy fats, and that not all fats are evil.

There are those fats which raise your risk of becoming diabetic, and other fats which don't need to be avoided. Some fats promote overweight and obesity, while others actually help improve your health. One fat may make your heart healthy while another fat can increase your risk of developing cardiovascular disease.

Let's look at the "good" and "bad" fats you need to familiarize yourself with so you know what you should and should not be eating to combat diabetes.

- **Good Fats** – These are monounsaturated and polyunsaturated fats, such as those found in plant oils like extra virgin olive oil and sunflower oil. Nuts and avocados, salmon, mackerel and other fish, flaxseeds and soy beans contain good fats.

- **Bad Fats** – These are saturated, hydrogenated and trans fats, and are found in cream, cheese and butter. They are often present in processed meat products like deli meats, and are ever-present in fast food, baked goods, highly processed foods, margarine and palm oil. Read your food labels and avoid foods and beverages that list saturated, hydrogenated or trans fats as ingredients.

One way to automatically consume good fats and avoid bad fats is to enjoy a plant-based diet.

Diabetics that eat predominantly unprocessed and minimally processed fresh fruits and vegetables, nuts and seeds will immediately limit the amount of unhealthy fat that enters their bodies.

We should mention that if you eat too much of any kind of fat you are not going to help your health. The good fats we just mentioned should be eaten in moderation, and you should strictly limit or totally remove bad fats from your diet.

What to Eat and What to Avoid

Let's address the elephant in the room regarding diabetes and food.

A lot of people think that a diabetes patient has to eat different foods than his friends or family members. ***This is entirely untrue.*** There are healthier choices which should be targeted, and unhealthier alternatives which should be limited.

When it comes right down to it though, if a diabetic person is exercising regularly, checking blood sugar levels constantly, getting plenty of restful sleep at night, staying hydrated and taking any prescribed medications, just about any food can be eaten on some occasions.

Having said that, there are foods which are recommended for preventing diabetes and which improve the experience for someone that has diabetes. There are also foods which should be avoided or limited. WebMD is a website dedicated to providing information you can use to become healthier. Here is a short list of some of the foods they recommend as good and bad choices for someone with diabetes.

- **Recommended Foods**

Whole grains like brown rice, quinoa, oatmeal, amaranth and millet. Sweet potatoes, all vegetables and fruits, and low-sodium veggies both canned and frozen if no sugar, syrup or other ingredients have been added.

Eat pasture-raised poultry and grass-fed beef, as well as wild-caught fish like salmon for protein and healthy fats. Eggs, nuts, seeds, natural spices and herbs, avocados and water. Drink herbal teas, black tea and coffee without sugar and cream.

- **Foods Which Should be Limited or Avoided**

Processed grains, especially white rice and white flour, as well as foods with lots of added sugar. Processed cereal, baked goods, fat-free foods, restaurant food and fast food, bottled fruit juices and energy drinks.

White bread, French fries and canned fruit with added sugar or syrup. Jams, jellies and preserves, gravies, and processed meats like hot dogs, sausage and bologna. Pork bacon, fried meats, cheese and dairy products, flavored coffees, beer and retail chocolate drinks.

The American Diabetes Association (ADA) reminds us that you can eat "bad food" from time to time. Just watch your portions and how regularly you decide to eat these types of foods.

The quickest way to avoid or treat diabetes and other significant health problems is to eat food that is as close to its natural state as possible. This means eating lots of fresh fruits and vegetables, nuts and seeds and whole grains which are not processed at all, or only processed a little bit.

When you shorten the path from nature to your dining room table, you have the best chance at being healthy. This means eating lots of leafy greens and other plant-based foods at most of your meals.

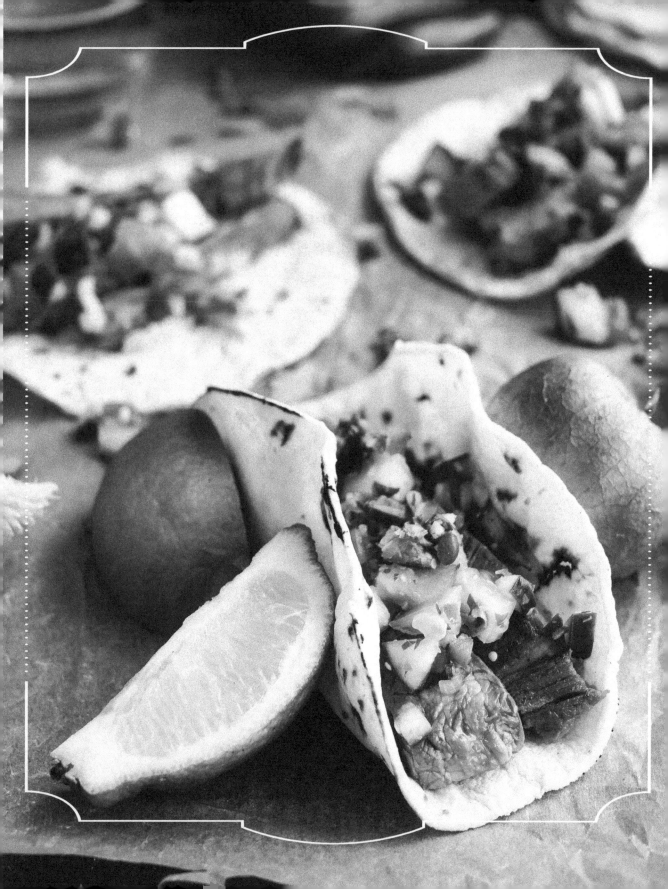

6

The Overlooked Importance of Staying Hydrated

Did you know the human body can go more than 30 days without eating anything? On the other hand, if you don't drink any water for just 3 days, a life-threatening situation can develop. This is how important it is for anyone to stay hydrated, especially someone who is prediabetic or diabetic.

Drink filtered water throughout the day. It varies from person to person, but the average water consumption for humans is about a gallon a day. This includes water in the beverages you drink, as well as the water contained in foods that you eat. Buy a BPA-free reusable water bottle and keep it with you so you can stay hydrated all day long.

Remember, water, herbal teas, black tea and coffee without sugar and cream are all recommended beverages for preventing and treating diabetes.

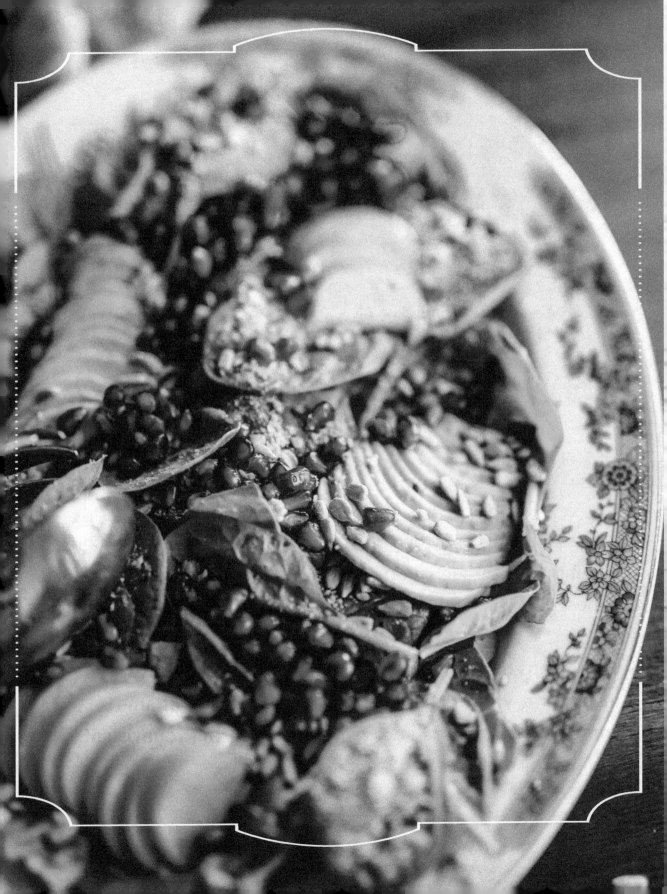

7

Stress Is a Cause (and Symptom) of Diabetes

Stress kills. The best friend of stress is inflammation. Stress causes inflammation throughout the body, and inflammation is present in almost every major disease and illness.

This means that if you constantly have a stressful presence in your life, you are increasing the risk that you inflame some body part or major organ, also increasing your risk of developing diabetes.

We have known for thousands of years that stress can be deadly. Chronic stress does not give your body and mind enough time to recuperate before another dose of stress lands on your plate. Sometimes we intentionally put ourselves in situations that are stressful. This is bad for a number of health reasons, and it doesn't help the person dealing with diabetes or trying to avoid diabetes.

Meditation and yoga has been used since ancient times to lower stress and anxiety. If you exercise regularly (and as you know, that is one of the recommendations for dealing with diabetes or keeping it from developing), you will naturally lower your stress level.

If you live in a highly toxic environment or a place where noise is constantly frustrating your eardrums, get out of those situations if you can.

Warm baths, green tea and aromatherapy are great stress relievers. Look at your life. Identify those situations and people or physical things that crank up your stress. Limit your exposure to them. Create a "quiet space" where you can retreat for mental peace and calmness. Limiting stress is important for treating diabetes, and the additional payoff is better mental and physical health overall.

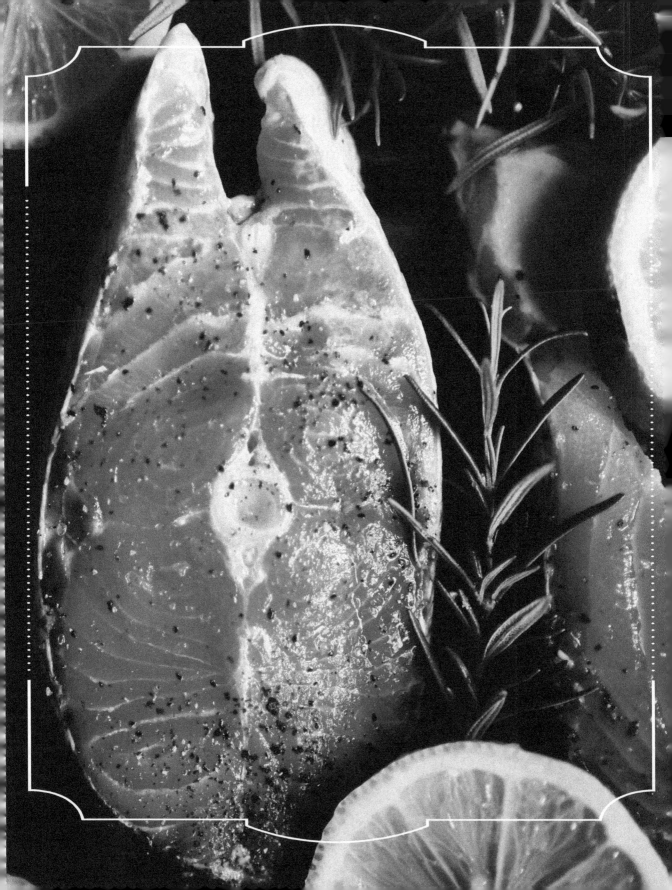

8

Assembling a Support Team

Remember earlier when we talked about how humans are social animals? You definitely need to assemble a team of people that help you de-stress and relax in social circles. You also need to develop a diabetes support team that includes health professionals and others so you can enjoy the best possible experience if you become diabetic.

Make a list of people that provide you a lot of joy emotionally and spiritually. Then add to that list any doctors, other caregivers, personal trainers, nutritionists and fitness experts you deal with. Include the names and contact information of these people, and don't forget to list your parents and children.

When you have a physical list written down that you can refer to, there is a greater chance that you will reach out to your diabetes support team for help when you need it. Write down a physical list of these individuals, print it out and have it laminated. Keep it with you wherever you go. Include a virtual list that you store on your smartphone, tablet and computer.

Don't be afraid to contact these people if you have questions, you need a shoulder to cry on, or you are excited about sharing some great piece of news because your health starts improving dramatically when you follow the health boosting advice in this report.

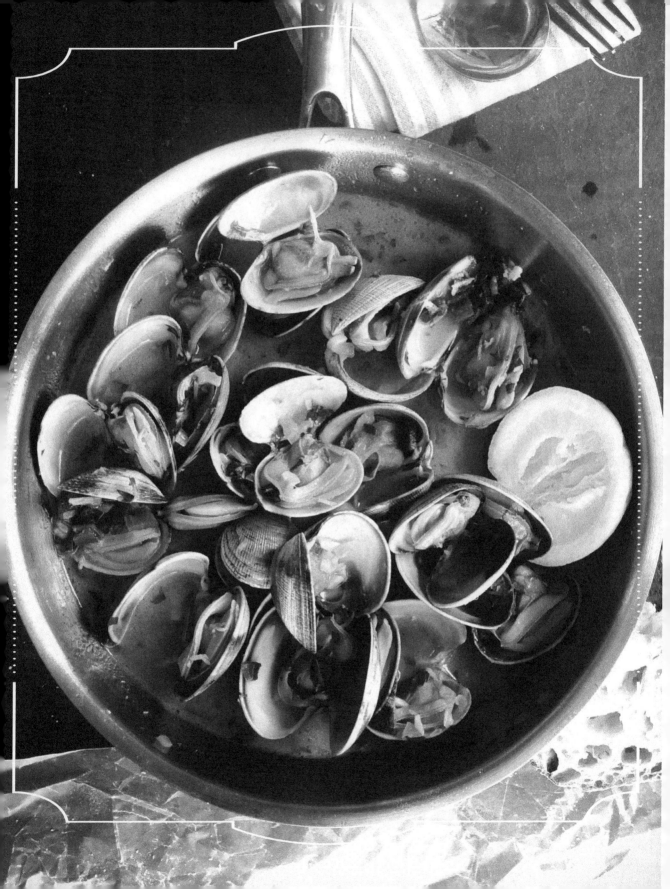

9

The 5 Words that Turn This Report Into Positive Results

The saying "knowledge is power" has been credited to a number of famous people. No matter who actually made that statement, it is partially correct. Before you take on any difficult task, you want to get all your facts together. You need to assemble relevant and applicable information that can help you achieve the desired result.

However, all the knowledge in the world will not help you if you don't do one simple thing.

You have to take action.

It is not at all exaggerating to say that the information in this report can save your life, if you remember those 5 words.

It can help you return to a high-energy, healthy and vibrant way of life, one that you may not have enjoyed in many years or even decades. Everything in this report can be done by just about anyone. You don't have to buy expensive or heavy exercise equipment, eating foods that lead to good health costs you less than foods that contribute to disease in the long run, and changing lifestyle behaviors doesn't cost athing.

These proven tips and best practices for preventing and reversing diabetes and treating diabetes have been proven to deliver nearly miraculous results for so many people just like you ... once they took action.

Get started today. The fact that you are reading this right now means you are serious about discovering just how healthy in mind and body you can possibly be. Whether you are prediabetic,

diabetic or interested in keeping this debilitating condition at bay by never experiencing it in the first place, the information in your report can help you realize the healthiest you.

Remember ...

1. Eat right. Use the do eat/don't eat list provided to guide your mealtime behaviors.

2. Get up and get moving as opposed to sitting and holding still. Get your 150 minutes of moderately intense physical activity each week.

3. Make any necessary lifestyle changes and minimize the amount of stress you experience.

You deserve to have a fulfilling, enjoyable and healthy life. Whether your goal is to prevent or treat diabetes, the information in this report can help you realize that dream existence, butonly if you heed these 5 words ... ***you have to take action.***

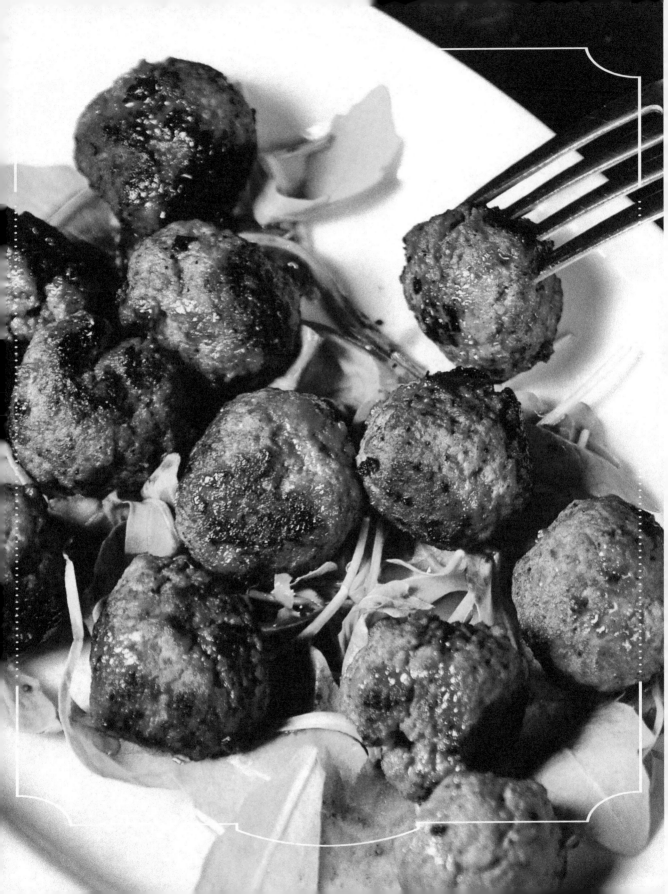

10

28-Day Meal Plan for People with Diabetes

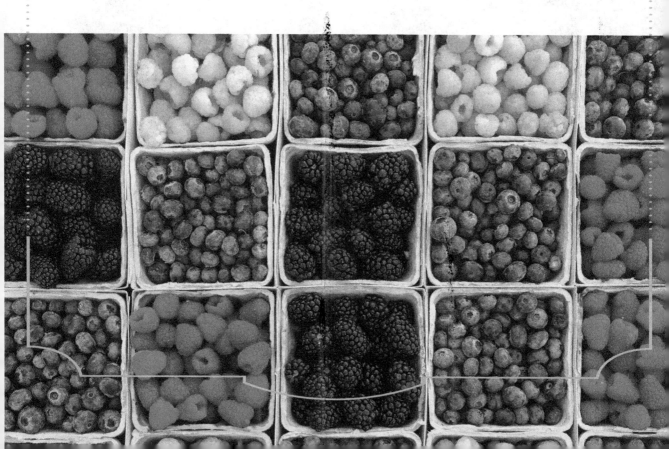

WEEK 1 - <u>Day 1</u>

Breakfast
- 2 (four-inch) whole grain pancakes
- 1/2 cup mixed berries
- 2 teaspoons sugar-free maple syrup
- 1 cup fat-free milk

Lunch
- Herbed Chicken Soup with Spring Vegetables [page 276]
- 1 cup tossed salad with 2 tablespoons low-calorie dressing
- 1 (one-ounce) whole grain roll
- 1 small apple

Dinner
- 4 ounces grilled salmon
- 1/2 cup brown rice cooked with low-fat chicken broth
- 1/2 cup cubed cucumber mixed with 1/2 cup cubed tomatoes tossed with 2 teaspoons olive oil and 1 teaspoon balsamic vinegar
- 5 roasted asparagus spears
- 1 (one-ounce) slice rye bread

Snacks

- 10 almonds
- 1/2 cup melon cubes tossed with 1 teaspoon lime juice

Today's Takeaway Tip: Fiber is extremely important for keeping blood sugar stable. Since fluctuating blood sugar levels can cause feelings of hunger, irritability and low energy, high-fiber foods, such as the whole grain pancakes, whole grain roll and brown rice, will help you to have a happier and healthier day.

Day 2

Breakfast

- 1/2 broiled grapefruit
- 1 ounce ready-to-eat whole grain cereal
- 1/2 cup fat-free milk

Lunch

- Cheese Melt: 2 ounces low-fat Cheddar cheese melted on 1 whole wheat English muffin with 2 slices tomato
- 1 serving Jicama Salad [page 278]
- 1 small peach

Dinner

- 3 ounces lean grilled flank steak
- 1/2 cup baked sweet potato with 1 teaspoon canola oil margarine
- 1/2 cup steamed spinach
- 1 cup romaine lettuce tossed with carrots, red peppers and 2 tablespoons low-calorie dressing
- 1/2 baked pear (halve and core unpeeled pear, place cut-side down in baking dish, pour low-cal cranberry juice halfway up the sides, bake in 375 degree oven for 30 to 40 minutes)

Snacks

- 1 cup sugar-free, low-fat yogurt
- 1 ounce whole grain crackers spread with 2 teaspoons reduced-fat peanut butter

Today's Takeaway Tip: Use non-hydrogenated spreads, like canola margarine, for your potatoes, breads and other foods instead of butter or regular margarine. Canola margarine has no trans fats, a contributing factor for heart disease of which people with diabetes are at risk for.

Day 3

Breakfast

- 1 slice whole wheat raisin bread spread with 1/4 cup part-skim ricotta cheese, toasted
- 1 slice (one-ounce) cooked Canadian bacon
- 1/2 cup mango slices

Lunch

- 3 ounces sliced turkey
- Mushroom Barley and Roasted Asparagus Salad [page 280]
- 1 small whole wheat pita bread
- 10 red grapes

Dinner

- 3 ounces baked cod
- 1 serving Grilled Ratatouille [page 282]
- 1/2 cup cooked whole wheat couscous
- 1 cup raw spinach tossed with 2 teaspoons olive oil and 2 teaspoons champagne vinegar
- 1/2 cup sugar-free, low-fat frozen yogurt

Snacks

- 1/2 cup cooked edamame
- 1 cup fat-free milk

Today's Takeaway Tip: Including more soy foods, like edamame, into your food plan may help lower cholesterol. High cholesterol plays a role in heart disease, a risk factor for people with diabetes.

Day 4

Breakfast

- Tropical Fruit Compote: 1/2 cup mixed pineapple, kiwi and papaya cubes
- 1 small toasted whole wheat pita bread
- 2 teaspoons sugarless jam
- 1 cup fat-free milk

Lunch

- White Bean Soup with Escarole [page 284]
- 1 slice multigrain bread
- 1 cup tossed salad with 2 teaspoons low-calorie dressing
- 1/2 cup (no added sugar) applesauce, sprinkled with cinnamon

Dinner

- 3 ounces grilled boneless pork loin chop
- 1/2 cup sautéed broccolini (sauté broccolini in 1 teaspoon olive oil)
- 1/2 cup roasted potatoes (leave peels on for extra fiber!)
- Angel Food Cake with Mangoes [page 286]

Snacks

- 1 ounce whole wheat pretzels
- 1 hard-boiled egg

Today's Takeaway Tip: Who says you can't have your cake and eat it too? For people with diabetes, desserts like Angel Food Cake can be a "yes," especially when it's paired with healthy vitamin C rich mangoes! Work with a registered dietitian to assist you in designing a plan that includes your favorite desserts.

Day 5

Breakfast

- 1 small (2-ounce) toasted whole wheat bagel papaya cubes

- 2 teaspoons reduced-fat cream cheese
- 2 slices tomato
- 1/2 cup sliced fresh strawberries
- 1/2 cup sugar-free, fat-free yogurt

Lunch

- Roast Beef Roll Up: 3 ounces lean roast beef rolled in a 10-inch whole wheat tortilla with 1/4 cup shredded carrots, 1 lettuce leaf and 1 tablespoon fat-free Ranch or Thousand Island dressing
- 1/2 cup red and yellow bell pepper strips
- 1 small peach

Dinner

- Grilled Chicken with Gremolata and Arugula Salad [page 288]
- 1/2 cup cooked whole wheat couscous
- 1/2 cup cooked zucchini and yellow squash (sauté in 1 teaspoon olive oil, sprinkle with 1/4 teaspoon dried oregano)
- 1 small orange, sliced

Snacks

- 1 (1/2-cup) serving sugar-free vanilla pudding
- 2 cups air-popped popcorn

> Today's Takeaway Tip: Choose your greens wisely — the darker the better. Arugula, for example, has nice dark leaves that provide ample amounts of antioxidants such as beta carotene and vitamin C. These antioxidants may have some heart protective values; good for people with diabetes!

Day 6

Breakfast

- 1/2 cup cooked sugar-free oatmeal, sprinkled with cinnamon
- 2 tablespoons raisins
- 1 cup fat-free milk

Lunch

- Halibut and Chickpea Salad [page 290]
- 1 ounce whole grain crackers
- 2 small plums

Dinner

- 1/2 grilled Cornish game hen
- 1/2 cup cooked wild rice
- 1/2 cup stir-fried broccoli with red bell pepper (stir-fry in 1 teaspoon canola oil in a wok over high heat)

- 1/2 cup mixed honeydew and cantaloupe chunks

Snacks
- 3 whole wheat graham crackers
- 1 frozen fruit bar (all fruit, no sugar added)

Today's Takeaway Tip: Make your diet full o'beans! The chickpeas added to the Halibut Salad are digested slowly, helping with good blood sugar control. In addition, beans offer an amazing protein value for the dollar, while lacking the artery-clogging fats and cholesterol of many other high-protein foods. cholesterol of many other high-protein foods.

Day 7

Breakfast
- 1 small bran muffin
- 1 teaspoon canola oil margarine
- 1/2 cup blueberries sprinkled with 1/2 teaspoon lemon zest
- 1 cup fat-free milk

Lunch
- Pizza Muffin: 1 small whole wheat English muffin topped with 1/2 cup marinara sauce, 1/4 cup part-skim mozzarella cheese,

- 1 ounce reduced- fat turkey pepperoni and 2 slices zucchini, broiled until cheese melts
- 1 cup tossed salad with 2 tablespoons low-calorie Italian dressing
- 2 tangerines

Dinner
- Grilled Tuna Steaks with Black Asian Sesame Crust [page 292]
- 1/2 cup cooked udon or soba noodles
- 1/2 cup stir-fried snow peas
- 1/2 cup mango sorbet

Snacks
- 6 ounces tomato juice
- 1 small whole wheat pita bread with 2 tablespoons hummus

Today's Takeaway Tip: Tuna, with its meaty texture and steak-like quality, is ideal as a substitute for red meats. Tuna contains high levels of omega-3 fatty acids which are known to lower high blood cholesterol, a risk factor for people with diabetes.

WEEK 2 - Day 8

Breakfast

- 1/2 recipe Blueberry Blast Smoothie [page 298]
- 1 slice (one-ounce) oatmeal bread
- 1 teaspoon canola margarine

Lunch

- Lentil and Rice Salad [page 144]
- Cherry Tomato and Zucchini Salad (1/2 cup each halved cherry tomatoes and zucchini cubes, drizzled with 2 teaspoons olive oil and 2 teaspoons balsamic vinegar)
- 1/2 cup fresh pineapple chunks

Dinner

- 4 ounces grilled scallops
- 1/2 cup cooked quinoa
- 1/2 cup sautéed red and yellow peppers with onion (sauté red and yellow bell pepper strips with thinly sliced red onion in 1 teaspoon olive oil, sprinkle with ½ teaspoon dried basil)
- 1/2 cup sliced grapes tossed with 1/2 cup sugar-free, fat-free vanilla yogurt

Snacks

- 1 ounce reduced-fat string cheese with 1 ounce whole grain crackers
- 1 cup low-fat, low-sodium vegetable soup

Today's Takeaway Tip: Berry nice! Blueberries are loaded with antioxidants — more than most other fruits. In addition, blueberries rank low on the glycemic index, an indicator on how carbohydrates effect blood sugar levels. Foods with lower scores raise blood sugar less.

Day 9

Breakfast

- 1 small whole wheat waffle
- 1 tablespoon sugar-free maple syrup
- 1 ounce reduced-fat turkey sausage link
- 1/2 banana

Lunch

- 3 ounces lean low-sodium ham slices
- Waldorf Salad [page 300]
- 1/2 toasted English muffin with 1 teaspoon canola margarine

Dinner

- Turkey Burgers with Tomato Corn Salsa [page 302]
- 1/2 cup sautéed spinach
- 1 cup cabbage salad (3/4 cup green or red cabbage with 1/4 cup shredded carrots, 2 tablespoons chopped onion and 1 tablespoon low- calorie dressing)

Snacks

- 1/2 small whole wheat toasted bagel with 2 teaspoons sugar-free jam
- 1 sugar-free, fat-free chocolate pudding

Today's Takeaway Tip: The apples in Waldorf Salad are high in a fiber called pectin. This "soluble" fiber contributes to reduced cholesterol levels and helps you to feel full longer. Choosing low-calorie foods that keep you satisfied contribute to good weight control, an issue for many people with diabetes.

Day 10

Breakfast

- 1/2 cup hot wheat cereal mixed with:
- 1/4 cup grated apple

- 2 tablespoons raisins
- 1 tablespoon sliced toasted almonds
- 1 cup fat-free milk

Lunch
- Chiken Tabbouleh Salad [page 304]
- 1 cup tossed salad (butter lettuce, carrots and cherry tomatoes, tossed with 2 tablespoons reduced-fat Thousand Island dressing)
- 1 nectarine

Dinner
- 4 ounces baked halibut fillet
- Garlicky Broccolini [page 308]
- 1 small (three-ounces) baked potato with 2 tablespoons reduced-fat sour cream and chopped chives
- 1/2 cup sugar-free, fat-free frozen chocolate yogurt

Snacks
- Salsa
- 1 ounce fat-free tortilla chips
- 1 ounce unsalted cashews

Day 11

Breakfast
- 1 serving Mixed Berry Fruit Salad [page 310]
- 1 (one-ounce) whole wheat roll
- 1 teaspoon canola margarine
- 1 cup fat-free milk

Lunch
- Manhattan Clam Chowder [page 312]
- 1 cup mixed field greens salad with 2 tablespoons fat-free blue cheese dressing
- 1 (one-ounce) slice seven-grain bread

Dinner
- Grilled Chicken with Tomato Cucumber Salad [page 316]

- 1/2 cup brown rice (cooked in low-fat, reduced-sodium chicken broth)
- 1/2 cup steamed snow peas
- 1/2 baked pear (halve and core unpeeled pear, place cut-side down in baking dish, pour low-cal cranberry juice 1/2 way up the sides, bake in 375 degree oven for 30 to 40 minutes)

Snacks
- 1/2 cup mango chunks
- 1/2 cup low-fat cottage cheese mixed with 1/2 teaspoon cinnamon and 1 teaspoon sugar-free jam

Today's Takeaway Tip: Great tasting food does not always require tons of salt, fat and sugar. Manhattan Clam Chowder is a good example of this — it tastes just as good as the cream-based version, but without the excess fat and calories.

Day 12

Breakfast
- Healthy Carrot Muffin [page 318]
- 1 ounce reduced-fat turkey sausage patty

- 1 cup fat-free milk

Lunch
- Tuna Pocket: (3 ounces canned tuna mixed with 2 tablespoons reduced- fat mayonnaise, 2 tablespoons each minced onion, celery and grated carrot), 1 romaine lettuce leaf, 1 ounce reduced-fat Swiss cheese, 1 small whole wheat pita bread
- 1/2 cup applesauce sprinkled with 1/2 teaspoon pumpkin pie spice

Dinner
- Sicilian-Style Cauliflower with Whole Wheat Pasta [page 320]
- 3 ounces grilled chicken
- 1 cup romaine lettuce tossed with tomatoes, zucchini and 2 tablespoons fat-free Caesar dressing
- 2 small plums

Snacks
- 1/2 apple with 1 tablespoon reduced-fat peanut butter
- 1 ounce whole wheat pretzels

Today's Takeaway Tip: Pasta took quite a beating during the low-carb craze. Truth is, a reasonable portion of whole wheat pasta, as prepared in Sicilian-Style Cauliflower with Whole Wheat Pasta, is high-fiber and filling; two pluses for people with diabetes. The key, as always, is portion size!

Day 13

Breakfast

- Yogurt Granola Parfait: (1 cup plain non-fat yogurt, layered with 1/2 cup sliced bananas and 1/4 cup low-fat granola)

Lunch

- Chicken and Pasta Soup [page 322]
- 1 ounce whole wheat crackers
- 1 cup tossed salad with watercress, sliced radishes and 2 tablespoons reduced-fat Italian dressing
- 3 whole wheat Fig Newton cookies

Dinner

- Linguine with Shrimp [page 324]
- 1/2 cup sautéed broccoli
- Mango Strawberry Snow Cones [page 326]

Snacks

- 6 ounces carrot juice
- 1 ounce whole wheat pita chips

Today's Takeaway Tip: Fill up on soup! High water content foods, such as soup, fruits and vegetables, help you feel full and satisfied and help prevent overeating. The Chicken and Pasta Soup delivers in many ways: lots of water in both broth and vegetables, low in fat and high in flavor.

Day 14

Breakfast

- Peach French Toast [page 327]
- 1 slice (one-ounce) Canadian bacon
- 1 cup fat-free milk

Lunch

- Greek Salad with Oregano Marinated Chicken [page 328]
- 1 ounce whole wheat breadsticks
- 1/2 cup fresh cherries

Dinner

- Crab Cakes [page 330]
- 1 small ear corn
- 1/2 cup sautéed kale(sauté in 1 teaspoon olive oil)
- 1/2 cup fresh raspberries topped with 2 tablespoons sugar-free, fat-free lemon yogurt

Snacks

- 2 ounces low-fat turkey slices rolled with 1 ounce reduced-fat Swiss cheese
- 1/2 cup sugar-free, fat-free tapioca pudding

Today's Takeaway Tip: Tired of the same old breakfast? Spice it up with a treat like Peach French Toast Bake — you actually might forget that you're eating healthy! It's important to know that you can have some treats, especially if you can tailor them to your needs.

WEEK 3 - <u>Day 15</u>

Breakfast

- Cheese and Tomato Omelet: (3 egg whites, 1/4 cup chopped tomato, 1/4 cup chopped mushrooms, 1 ounce reduced-fat Swiss cheese cooked in 1 teaspoon canola margarine or olive oil)
- 1 (one-ounce) slice pumpernickel bread
- 1/2 cup fresh blackberries

Lunch

- Poached Salmon with Lemon Mint Tzatziki [page 332]
- 3 whole wheat sesame breadsticks
- 1/2 cup sliced peaches with mint sprig

Dinner

- Thaini Edamame Burger [page 180]
- 1 small (2-ounce) whole wheat toasted bun
- 1 cup red leaf lettuce salad tossed with 1/2 cup diced cucumber, 1/2 sliced tomato and 1/4 cup shredded carrots with 2 tablespoons non-fat French dressing

Snack

- 2 small fresh apricots
- 1 cup fat-free milk

Today's Takeaway Tip: You'll see yogurt throughout this 30-day menu planner. It's a wonderful source of calcium, high in protein and can substitute for cream and other high-fat ingredients. Used in the Poached Salmon with Lemon Tzatziki, it makes a creamy, satisfying sauce to the salmon without all the fat of other sauces.

Day 16

Breakfast

- Apple Muffins [page 336]
- 1/2 cup fat-free cottage cheese sprinkled with 1/4 teaspoon cinnamon

Lunch

- Vegetarian Sandwich: (3 tablespoons hummus, 2 slices tomato, 1/4 cup shredded carrots, 2 thin slices cucumber, 2 slices whole wheat bread)
- 1/2 cup reduced-sodium, low-fat vegetable soup
- 1/2 cup cantaloupe cubes with lime wedge

Dinner

- Baked Mahi Mahi with Wine and Herbs [page 338]
- 1/2 cup roasted red potatoes
- 1/2 cup broiled eggplant
- 1/2 cup sliced papaya

Snacks

- Toasted Pita Triangles [page 301]
- 1 ounce part-skim string cheese

Today's Takeaway Tip: Go vegetarian! By eating naturally low-in-fat vegetarian foods like beans and grains, you can slash your saturated fat content while adding tons of fiber to your diet. Foods like hummus provide a rich taste without guilt.

Day 17

Breakfast

- 1/2 cup cooked oatmeal sprinkled with 1/4 teaspoon each cinnamon and nutmeg
- 1/2 sliced banana
- 1 cup fat-free milk

Lunch

- Minestrone Soup with Pasta, Beans and Vegetables [page 340]
- 1 cup romaine lettuce, 1 teaspoon Parmesan cheese, 1/2 cup halved cherry tomatoes tossed with 2 tablespoons non-fat Caesar dressing
- 1 (one-ounce) sliced whole wheat Italian bread
- 3 dried apricot halves

Dinner

- Crispy Chicken Tenders [page 188]
- Coleslaw: (1/2 cup shredded green cabbage, 1/4 cup shredded carrots, 2 tablespoons minced red onion, 1/2 teaspoon poppy seeds tossed with 2 teaspoons olive oil and 2 teaspoons apple cider vinegar)
- 1/2 small baked potato topped with 1 tablespoon tomato salsa
- 1/2 cup sugar-free, fat-free frozen peach yogurt

Snack

- 1 ounce shelled walnuts
- 1 rice cake spread with 2 teaspoons sugar-free raspberry jam

> Today's Takeaway Tip: If you love the taste of fried foods, but can't afford the calories and fat, learn the art of substitution. Crispy Chicken Tenders, which is cereal-coated and baked, gives the texture of fried chicken without the risk of added pounds!

Day 18

Breakfast
1 small whole wheat muffin
1 teaspoon canola margarine
1/2 cup sugar-free, fat-free lemon yogurt topped with 1/2 cup raspberries

Lunch:
Slow-Roasted Salmon with Cucumber Dill Salad [page 344]
1/2 toasted English muffin
1 peeled and sliced kiwi

Dinner
- Thai Shrimp Stir-Fry with Tomatoes and Basil [page 348]
- 1 all-fruit frozen juice bar

Snacks

1/2 apple spread with 2 teaspoons reduced-fat peanut butter

1 ounce baked low-fat tortilla chips with 2 tablespoons salsa

Today's Takeaway Tip: Kiwi is an excellent source of vitamin C (an important antioxidant that may prevent heart disease), fiber and potassium. In fact, kiwis supply more potassium than a medium banana!

Day 19

Breakfast

- Open Faced Egg and Tomato Sandwich: (1 poached egg, 1 slice tomato, 1 slice cooked Canadian bacon or 1 {one-ounce} slice turkey)
- 1/2 toasted whole wheat English muffin
- 1/2 cup fresh poached figs (simmer figs in equal parts apple juice and water, seasoned with a cinnamon stick and clove or two until soft, serve with poaching liquid)
- 1 cup fat-free milk

Lunch

- 1 cup low-fat, low-sodium black bean soup topped with

- 1 tablespoon low- fat sour cream
- 4 baked tortilla chips
- 1/2 cup carrot sticks dipped in 1 tablespoon non-fat Ranch dressing

1/2 cup water-packed mandarin oranges

Dinner
- Snapper with Grape Tomatoes and Mushrooms [page 350]
- 1/2 cup cooked whole wheat couscous
- Spinach salad: (1 cup spinach leaves, 2 slices red onion, 1/4 cup sliced mushrooms, 1 tablespoon sliced toasted almonds and 2 tablespoons non- fat Italian salad dressing)
- 3 sugar-free vanilla sandwich crème cookies

Snack
2 tablespoons Chunky Guacamole with 1 ounce whole wheat crackers [page 198]

1 cup plain non-fat yogurt mixed with 2 teaspoons sugar-free strawberry jam

Today's Takeaway Tip: While watching your quantity of fat is important, it is equally important to look at the quality. The avocados in the Chunky Guacamole are an excellent source of monounsaturated fat, the type that is good for your cholesterol. Moreover, the avocado is a source of lutein, a phytochemical that seems to help prevent age-related macular degeneration. This may be important for people with diabetes who may have eye problems associated with the disease.

Day 20

Breakfast

- 1 ounce Shredded Wheat Cereal
- 1 ounce cooked turkey bacon
- 1/2 cup blueberries
- 1/2 cup fat-free milk

Lunch

- Chopped Nicoise Salad [page 354]
- 1 small whole grain roll with 1 teaspoon canola oil margarine
- 1/2 cup (no sugar added) applesauce with 1/4 teaspoon ground ginger, served warm

Dinner

- Chicken Cacciatore [page 356]
- 1/2 cup whole wheat fusilli pasta
- 1/2 cup sautéed broccolini topped with 1 tablespoon toasted pine nuts
- 1/2 peach sprinkled with 2 teaspoons unsweetened toasted coconut

Snacks

- Hot Chocolate [page 360]
- 1 ounce whole wheat pretzels dipped in Dijon mustard

Today's Takeaway Tip: Decadent foods like chocolate are not off limits. The creamy Hot Chocolate is a perfect example of a how to enjoy a small amount of a rich food that is normally taboo. When combined with low-fat milk and bolstered with spices, chocolate is just a sip away.

Day 21

Breakfast

- 2 (four-inch) whole wheat pancakes topped with 1/4 cup part-skim ricotta cheese mixed with 2 teaspoons sugar-free blueberry jam
- 1 vegetarian sausage link
- 1/2 cup fat-free milk

Lunch

- Chickpea and Spinach Salad with Cumin Dressing [page 362]
- 1 toasted small whole wheat tortilla
- 1/2 cup each red and yellow pepper strips
- 1/2 cup water-packed canned pineapple

Dinner

- San Francisco Cioppino [page 364]
- 1 (one-ounce) slice whole wheat sourdough bread
- 1 cup butter lettuce salad with 1/4 cup diced zucchini, 1/4 cup diced yellow tomato, 1/4 cup diced carrot, 2 teaspoons gorgonzola cheese, tossed with 2 tablespoons non-fat blue cheese dressing
- 1 small baked apple baked in low-calorie cranberry juice cocktail

Snacks

- 1/2 small baked sweet potato topped with 2 teaspoons sugar-free maple syrup
- 1 ounce reduced-fat Cheddar cheese wedge

Today's Takeaway Tip: It was once believed that to control high cholesterol you should eliminate shellfish. Research has shown that it is actually foods high in saturated fat, not dietary cholesterol, that effect blood cholesterol. Shellfish (in San Francisco Cioppino) are actually very low in saturated fat and total fat. In addition, clams, shrimp, squid and crab are excellent sources of B12, potassium and iron.

WEEK 4 - Day 22

Breakfast

- 1/2 serving Applegurt [page 366]
- 1 scrambled egg cooked in 1 teaspoon olive oil, topped with 1 teaspoon chopped chives

Lunch

- Raspberry Chicken Salad [page 368]
- 1/2 whole wheat bagel spread with 2 teaspoons reduced-fat cream cheese
- 1 orange

Dinner

- 4 ounces grilled beef tenderloin
- Oven Baked Garlic [page 216]
- 5 grilled asparagus spears
- Mixed Tomato Salad: (1/2 cup cubed red tomatoes, 1/4 cup halved cherry tomatoes, 2 tablespoons chopped Vidalia onion, 2 teaspoons minced fresh basil drizzled with 2 teaspoons balsamic vinegar)
- 10 red grapes

Snacks

- 1 ounce roasted unsalted cashews
- 1/2 cup edamame

Today's Takeaway Tip: Instead of frying, try baking. Oven Baked Garlic are a perfect example of how to enjoy the crunch of fried foods without all the excess fat and calories.

Day 23

Breakfast
- Pumpkin Muffins [page 372]
- 1 cup fat-free milk

Lunch
- Crab Salad Sandwich: (mix 3 ounces cooked crabmeat with 1 tablespoon low-fat mayonnaise, 1/4 cup chopped red pepper, 1/4 cup chopped celery, 1/2 teaspoon capers; place in a whole wheat pita pocket with spinach or lettuce leaves.)
- 1/2 cup reduced-sodium, low-fat tomato soup
- 1/2 cup sugar-free, fat-free vanilla pudding

Dinner
- Garlic Lime Chicken with Olives [page 374]
- 1/2 cup cooked whole wheat orzo
- 1/2 cooked artichoke dipped in 1 tablespoon low-fat mayonnaise mixed with 1/4 teaspoon lemon zest
- 2 plums

Snack
- 1/2 banana spread with 1 teaspoon almond butter

- 6 ounces sugar-free, fat-free blueberry yogurt

Today's Takeaway Tip: Pumpkin boasts an impressive amount of beta carotene, a healthy antioxidant that may help prevent disease. Canned pumpkin, used in Pumpkin Muffins, is just as nutritious as raw.

Day 24

Breakfast
- 1 egg fried in 1 teaspoon olive oil
- 1 (one-ounce) slice rye bread
- 1/2 cup sliced strawberries mixed with 1/2 cup plain yogurt

Lunch
- Pumpernickel Tes Sandwich [page 376]
- 1/2 cup each blanched broccoli and cauliflower dipped in 2 tablespoons non-fat blue cheese dressing
- 1 small orange

Dinner
- Pork Au Poivre [page 378]
- 1/2 cup sautéed spinach

- 1 cup tossed salad with 2 tablespoons non-fat Thousand Island dressing
- Ginger Tea Cake [page 380]

Snacks

- 1/2 cup pomegranate seeds
- 1 ounce whole wheat pretzels

Today's Takeaway Tip: Pomegranates are very high in vitamin C, potassium and fiber and low in calories. They also contain tannins, anthocyanins and ellagic acids, three important antioxidants that may help prevent heart disease. Look for pomegranates from September through February.

Day 25

Breakfast

- 1/2 cup hot seven-grain cereal
- 1/4 cup chopped dried apples
- 1 cup fat-free milk

Lunch

- Chicken Kebabs [page 382]
- 1 small whole wheat pita bread, warmed
- 1/2 cup sautéed portobello mushrooms (cook in 1 teaspoon olive oil)
- 10 green grapes

Dinner

- 3 ounces grilled salmon
- Grilled Salad with Herbed Vinaigrette [page 384]
- 1/2 cup brown rice cooked in reduced-sodium chicken broth
- 1 serving Banana Cream Pie [page 386]

Snack

- 1 hard-boiled egg
- 6 ounces low-sodium tomato juice

Today's Takeaway Tip: It's important to keep all kinds of textures in your food plan. This low-calorie, low-fat Banana Cream Pie's smooth creamy texture and crisp crust will make your taste buds happy, but keep your waistline trim.

Day 26

Breakfast
Strawberry and Tofu Smoothie [page 387]
1 rice cake with 2 teaspoons cashew butter

Lunch
- Chilli Bean Soup With Avocado [page 388]
- 1/2 cup sliced English cucumber and1/2 cup halved grape tomatoes drizzled with 2 teaspoons balsamic vinegar
- 3 whole wheat sesame breadsticks
- 4 dried plums

Dinner
- 3 ounces baked tilapia
- Seared Greens with Red Onion and Vinegar [page 390]
- 1/2 cup barley cooked in reduced-sodium chicken broth
- 1 cup tossed salad drizzled with 1 teaspoon walnut oil and 2 teaspoons herb vinegar
- 1/2 cup sliced bananas topped with 1 tablespoon lite whipped topping

Snacks

- 1/2 cup water-packed mixed fruit salad
- 1/2 cup low-fat cottage cheese with 1 tablespoon toasted slivered almonds

Today's Takeaway Tip: Think dark when it comes to choosing your greens. Light colored greens like iceberg lettuce provide little nutrition. The chard used in Seared Greens with Red Onion and Vinegar is full of fiber, beta carotene and iron.

Day 27

Breakfast

- 1/2 whole wheat bagel with 1 ounce melted reduced-fat Jarlsberg cheese
- 1/2 cup sliced star fruit (also known as carambola)

Lunch

- 3 ounces grilled shrimp
- Roasted Beet & Mandarin Orange Salad [page 392]
- 1 small whole grain roll
- 1 teaspoon canola margarine

Dinner

- Spaghetti with Swiss Chard and Pecorino Cheese [page 394]
- Pimiento Green [page 398]
- 1/2 cup sugar-free, fat-free frozen vanilla yogurt

Snacks

- 2 cups air-popped popcorn
- 1 ounce lean turkey breast

Today's Takeaway Tip: Beets are low in calories and provide significant amounts of folate (helpful in the prevention of heart disease), vitamin C and potassium.

The carbohydrate count of beets is higher than many other vegetables, but beets are perfectly acceptable for a person with diabetes. Go ahead and enjoy the Beet and Mandarin Orange Salad, guilt-free.

Day 28

Breakfast

- 3 scrambled egg whites (scramble in 1 teaspoon olive oil, top with 1 tablespoon reduced-fat Cheddar cheese and 1 teaspoon chopped basil)

- Blueberry Sauce [page 399]
- 1 cup fat-free milk

Lunch

- Open Face Lean Roast Beef Sandwich: (3 ounces lean roast beef, 1 romaine lettuce leaf, 1 slice tomato, 2 teaspoons Dijon honey mustard, 1 slice whole grain bread) Carrot, Carrot Green Apple Mint Salad [page 246]

Dinner

- Tofu and Vegetable Stir-Fry [page 248]
- 1/2 cup cooked soba noodles
- 1/2 cup honeydew chunks sprinkled with 1 teaspoon lemon juice and 1 teaspoon minced crystallized ginger

Snacks

- 2 tablespoons low-fat bean dip with 1 ounce baked tortilla chips
- 6 ounces sugar-free, non-fat raspberry yogurt

Today's Takeaway Tip: Tofu adds a wonderful vegetarian option for your meal plan that's low in saturated fat and high in protein. One of the great things about tofu is its ability to absorb whatever flavors you add — in Tofu and vegetables Stir-Fry, the tofu takes on an Asian flavor.

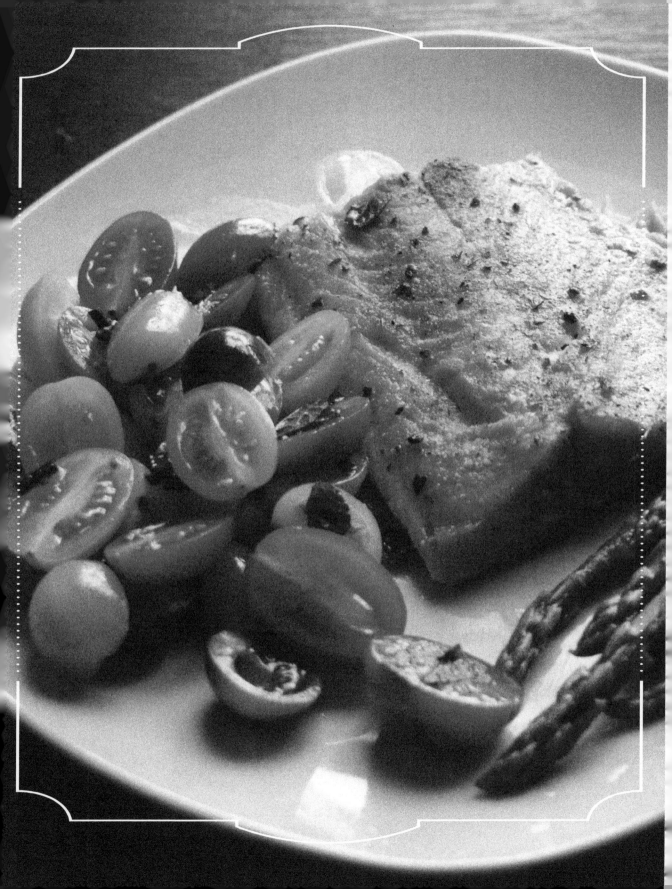

HERBED CHICKEN SOUP WITH SPRING VEGETABLES

Prep Time: 20 minutes | Cook Time: 25 minutes | Yield: 4 servings

Ingredients

3 sprigs + 1 tbsp fresh flat-leaf parsley, chopped

3 sprigs + 1 tbsp fresh tarragon, chopped

3 sprigs fresh thyme

1 bay leaf

1 small onion, chopped

2 medium carrots, sliced

1 stalk celery, sliced

3 long strips lemon zest

4 bone-in chicken breast halves, skin removed (2½ to 3 lb)

4 cups chicken broth, low-sodium canned or homemade

1 bunch medium asparagus, thick ends trimmed, cut into 1-inch segments

⅓ cup fresh or frozen peas

5 medium shiitake mushrooms, stemmed and sliced

DIRECTIONS

1. Tie the parsley, tarragon, and thyme sprigs and bay leaf together with kitchen twine and put in a large saucepan with the onion, carrot, celery, lemon zest, and chicken breasts.
2. Cover with the broth, bring just to a boil over high heat, skim off any foam that comes to the surface.
3. Adjust the heat to very low and cover.
4. Cook the chicken until firm to the touch, about 20 minutes.
5. Remove the chicken to a platter, when cool enough to handle and pull into large strips; discard the bones.
6. When ready to serve, add the asparagus, peas, and mushrooms to the broth.
7. Cook until the vegetables are just tender, about 3 to 5 minutes, and remove herb bundle.
8. Return chicken to the broth and warm through.
9. Divide chicken between 4 large soup bowls and ladle some broth and vegetables into each bowl.
10. Garnish each soup with the chopped parsley and tarragon.
11. Serve.

Per Servings:

269 Calories | 4g Fat | 1g Saturated Fat | 47g Protein | 14g Carbs | 5g Fiber

JICAMA SALAD

Cook Time: 25 minutes | Yield: 4 servings

Ingredients

1 large jícama, peeled and thinly sliced

1 small red onion, peeled and thinly sliced

2 Tbsp finely chopped cilantro

2 Tbsp finely chopped mint

3 Tbsp lime juice

1 Tsp salt

DIRECTIONS

1. Arrange jicama and red onion slices on a serving plate.
2. Sprinkle with salt, lime juice, mint, and cilantro.

TIPS

Jícama looks like a turnip or a large radish with brown skin.

Look for jícama that are firm with dry roots and not bruised or flawed. Peel skin before eating or cooking

MUSHROOM BARLEY AND ROASTED ASPARAGUS SALAD

Prep Time: 20 minutes | Cook Time: 40 minutes | Yield: 4 servings

Ingredients

3/4 cup pearl barley rinsed

2 tablespoon sprigs fresh thyme plus 1minced leaves

3 cup stems fresh flat-leaf parsley plus 1/3chopped leaves

1 Bay Leaf

2 in lemons zest peeledlarge strips

10 ounces button mushrooms trimmed and thinly sliced (about 4 cups)

1/3 cup freshly squeezed lemon juice

2 teaspoons kosher salt

2 teaspoons dijon mustard

Freshly ground black pepper

1/3 cup extra virgin olive oil plus more for cooking the asparagus

1/2 medium shallot minced

2 bunches medium asparagus woody stems trimmed (about 2 pounds)

DIRECTIONS

1. Put the barley in a medium pot with water to cover by a few inches and salt it generously. Tie the thyme sprigs, parsley stems, and bay leaf together with a piece of kitchen twine and add to the pot, along with the lemon peel. Simmer, stirring occasionally, until tender, about 30 minutes. Drain and remove the herbs and lemon.

2. Meanwhile, toss the mushrooms with 2 tablespoons of the lemon juice and 1/2 teaspoon of the salt in a large bowl. Whisk the remaining lemon juice with the mustard, remaining salt, and pepper, to taste, In a small bowl. Gradually whisk in the olive oil, starting with a few drops and then adding the rest in a steady stream to make a smooth, slightly thick vinaigrette. Add the shallots.

3. Toss the mushrooms, barley, and the dressing together. Stir in the chopped herbs. Set aside at room temperature for about 1 hour for the flavors to come together.

4. Preheat the oven to 450 degrees F.

5. Spread the spears in a single layer in a shallow baking pan, drizzle with olive oil, sprinkle with salt, and roll to coat thoroughly. Roast the asparagus until lightly browned and tender, about 10 minutes, giving the pan a good shake about halfway through. Serve.

GRILLED RATATOUILLE

Prep Time: 20 minutes | Cook Time: 30 minutes | Yield: 4 servings

Ingredients

1 head garlic

olive oil, for brushing vegetables

3 large tomatoes, cored and halved crosswise

1 small Eggplant, cut into 1-inch-thick rounds

2 large bell peppers, cored, halved and seeded

2 medium zucchini, halved lengthwise

1 cup canned Chickpeas, drained and rinsed

2 Tbs. chopped fresh basil

1/2 cup tomato sauce, option

DIRECTIONS

1. Preheat gas grill to medium or prepare charcoal fire
2. Using sharp knife, slice off upper third from garlic head. Place garlic head in sheet of aluminum foil, sprinkle with oil and loosely wrap. Place on fairly hot section of grill and let cook while grilling vegetables, about 30 minutes.

3. Brush surfaces of tomato halves with oil and place on grill, skin side down. Brush Eggplant slices with oil and place on grill. Trim white ribs from peppers; brush with oil and place on grill, along with halved zucchini. (If there's not enough room, grill vegetables in stages.) Sprinkle all vegetables with salt and pepper to taste

4. Grill vegetables, sans tomatoes, using tongs to turn frequently, until tender but not overly charred.

5. When bell peppers are done, transfer to medium bowl, cover with plastic wrap and set aside for 10 minutes.

6. Transfer remaining vegetables to large, shallow, casserole dish.

7. Scrape and discard charred skin from bell peppers.

8. Coarsely chop all vegetables and transfer to large saucepan. Add Chickpeas, basil, and salt and pepper to taste.

9. Remove garlic from foil, squeeze out several individual cloves and chop or mash. Add to vegetables and mix well. (Save remaining roasted garlic for another use.)

10. Over medium-low heat, gently heat ratatouille, stirring often and adding a little tomato sauce to moisten if desired. Serve with grilled polenta slices.

WHITE BEAN SOUP WITH ESCAROLE

Prep Time: 15 minutes | Cook Time: 35 minutes | Yield: 8 servings

Ingredients

1 tablespoon olive oil

1 small onion, chopped

5 garlic cloves, minced

3 cans (14-1/2 ounces each) reduced-sodium chicken broth

1 can (14-1/2 ounces) diced tomatoes, undrained

1/2 teaspoon Italian seasoning

1/4 teaspoon crushed red pepper flakes

1 cup uncooked whole wheat orzo pasta

1 bunch escarole or spinach, coarsely chopped (about 8 cups)

1 can (15 ounces) cannellini beans, rinsed and drained

1/4 cup grated Parmesan cheese

DIRECTIONS

1. In a Dutch oven, heat oil over medium heat. Add onion and garlic; cook and stir until tender. Add broth, tomatoes, Italian seasoning and pepper flakes; bring to a boil. Reduce heat; simmer, uncovered, 15 minutes.

2. Stir in orzo and escarole. Return to a boil; cook 12-14 minutes or until orzo is tender. Add beans; heat through, stirring occasionally. Sprinkle servings with cheese.

3. Freeze option: Freeze cooled soup in freezer containers. To use, partially thaw in refrigerator overnight. Heat through in a saucepan, stirring occasionally and adding a little broth if necessary.

Per Servings (1 cup soup with 1-1/2 teaspoons cheese):
174 Calories | 3g Fat | 1g Saturated Fat | 2mg Cholesterol | 572mg sodium | 28g carbohydrate (3g sugars, 8g fiber) | 9g protein

ANGEL FOOD CAKE WITH MANGOES

Prep Time: 15 minutes | Cook Time: 10 minutes | Yield: 8 servings

Ingredients

1 Angel food cake

Strawberries fresh

2 Mangoes

1 Cup Sugar

5 Tablespoons Lime Juice

2 Teaspoons Corn Starch

1 Tablespoon Water

Can a Diabetic Eat Angel Food Cake?

As a type 2 diabetic, you can eat angel food cake in moderate amounts, but a serving should replace a serving of milk, starch or fruit.

DIRECTIONS

1. Puree the mangoes until smooth.
2. Pour into a saucepan and heat over medium heat.
3. Add lime juice and sugar.
4. Stir together water and cornstarch.
5. Slowly stir the cornstarch mixture into the mango mixture.
6. Heat until slightly thickening and remove from heat.
7. Let cool a little and then place in the fridge to chill.
8. Slice the cake, strawberries and then serve with sauce.

GRILLED CHICKEN WITH GREMOLATA AND ARUGULA

Prep Time: 20 minutes | Cook Time: 25 minutes | Yield: 4 servings

Ingredients

1 gallon water

1 cup kosher salt

1 Tbsp. coriander seed

1 Tbsp. whole black pepper

1 Tbsp. mustard seed

1 Tbsp. fennel seed

1 bay leaf

1 sprig fresh thyme

1 (2½ lb.) whole chicken, back bone removed and butterflied

1 Tbsp. lemon zest

1 Tbsp. orange zest

1 Tbsp. freshly squeezed lemon juice

1 Tbsp. garlic, minced fine

¼ cup parsley leaves, minced fine

1 tsp. fresh mint, minced fine

½ cup extra virgin olive oil

Kosher salt, to taste

DIRECTIONS

1. In a large pot combine water, salt, coriander seed, black pepper, mustard seed, fennel seed, bay leaf and thyme.
2. Bring to a boil, then remove from heat and let steep for 1 hour.
3. Strain and chill brine to below 40°F before adding chicken.
4. Brine chicken for at least 6 hours or overnight in the refrigerator.
5. Remove chicken from brine and pat dry before grilling.
6. Grill chicken over indirect heat until juices run clear and the skin is golden brown and delicious (internal temperature should be 150°F).
7. Remove chicken from heat and cover with foil.
8. Let rest for 15 minutes before carving.
9. Chicken can be served warm or at room temperature.
10. For the gremolata, combine zests, lemon juice, garlic, parsley, mint, olive oil and salt in a bowl.
11. Spoon desired amount of gremolata over chicken

HALIBUT AND CHICKPEA SALAD

Prep Time: 20 minutes | Cook Time: 8 minutes | Yield: 1 servings

Ingredients

Halibut:

1 (6-ounce) halibut steak

2 teaspoons extra-virgin olive oil

1/4 teaspoon salt

1/4 teaspoon freshly ground black pepper

Salad:

1 head frisee, chopped

1 cup arugula, chopped

10 cherry tomatoes, halved

1 (15-ounce) can chickpeas (garbanzo beans)

1 fennel bulb, stalk removed, halved, and thinly sliced

1/4 cup extra-virgin olive oil

1 lemon, juiced

2 teaspoons honey

Ingredients

1 teaspoon ground cumin

1/2 teaspoon salt

1/2 teaspoon freshly ground black pepper

DIRECTIONS

1. For the halibut: Place a grill pan over medium-high heat. Brush the halibut with olive oil and season both sides with salt and pepper. Grill until cooked through, about 4 minutes per side.

2. For the salad: In a large bowl, combine the frisee, arugula, tomatoes, chickpeas, and fennel. In a small bowl mix together the olive oil, lemon juice, honey, cumin, salt, and pepper. Drizzle the olive oil mixture over the salad and toss to combine. Serve with fish.

3. Cooking Tip: Again, feel free to modify the recipe as needed for your household. I am not strict about amounts of veggies in the salad – I usually throw in a couple handfuls of arugula, chop up some frisee, throw in some tomatoes, add sugar snap peas for crunch, use only about 1/4 of a fennel bulb (the flavor is great but can be overpowering), and use only half a can of chickpeas. So, so good.

GRILLED TUNA STEAKS WITH ASIAN SESAME CRUST

Prep Time: 10 minutes | Cook Time: 6 minutes |

Marinate 20 minutes | Yield: 4 servings

Ingredients

1/2 cup low-sodium soy sauce

1/4 cup scallions (chopped, white and light green parts)

2 tablespoons fresh lemon juice

1 teaspoon sesame oil

1 teaspoon fresh ginger (grated)

4 (6-ounce) tuna steaks

1/2 cup sesame seeds (white and black combined or white only)

1/2 teaspoon cornstarch

DIRECTIONS

1. Gather the ingredients
2. In a large zip-top bag, combine the soy sauce, chopped scallions, lemon juice, sesame oil, and fresh ginger. Swish everything around in the bag until it's well combined.
3. Add the tuna steaks, turning within the bag to coat them

3. completely with the marinade. Press the excess air out of the bag, seal, and marinate in the refrigerator for about 20 minutes. Preheat a countertop contact grill to "sear" or the highest temperature setting, or preheat an open grill pan over high heat.

4. Place the sesame seeds on a plate or a shallow dish. Remove the tuna steaks from the marinade bag, brushing the scallions off the steaks and reserving the marinade. One at a time, coat the steaks in sesame seeds on all sides, pressing the seeds into the steak so they'll stick.

5. Spray the grill plates lightly with nonstick spray and place the steaks on the grill, closing the cover so the top grill rests evenly on the steaks. Do not press down. Grill for about 3 minutes for a rare, pink interior. Grill longer if you prefer your tuna cooked through. Remove from the grill and keep warm.

6. If you are using an open grilling surface, carefully flip the tuna steaks with a pair of tongs after 3 minutes and cook for 3 minutes on the other side.

7. While the tuna cooks, pour the marinade into a small saucepan and bring to a boil. Add the cornstarch, stirring with a whisk. Simmer for about 3 to 4 minutes, until the sauce thickens.

8. Serve.

BLUEBERRY BLAST SMOOTHIE

Prep Time: 5 minutes | Cook Time: - minutes | Yield: 4 servings

Ingredients

1/2 cup light vanilla ice cream

1/2 cup frozen blueberries

3 ounces raspberry or blueberry low-fat yogurt

1/4 cup low-fat milk, or soy milk

DIRECTIONS

Add all the ingredients to a blender or small food processor and mix until well blended. Pour into a glass and enjoy!

Nutritional Information

Calories 276

Calories from Fat 18%

Protein 9.7 g

Carbohydrates 48.2 g

Dietary fiber 2.3 g

Fat 5.7 g

Saturated fat 3.2 g

Cholesterol 26.9 mg

Sodium 133 mg

Sugars 42.5 g

Calcium 329 mg

Vitamin C 3.4 mg

Iron 0.4 mg

Potassium 455 mg

Vitamin A 526 I

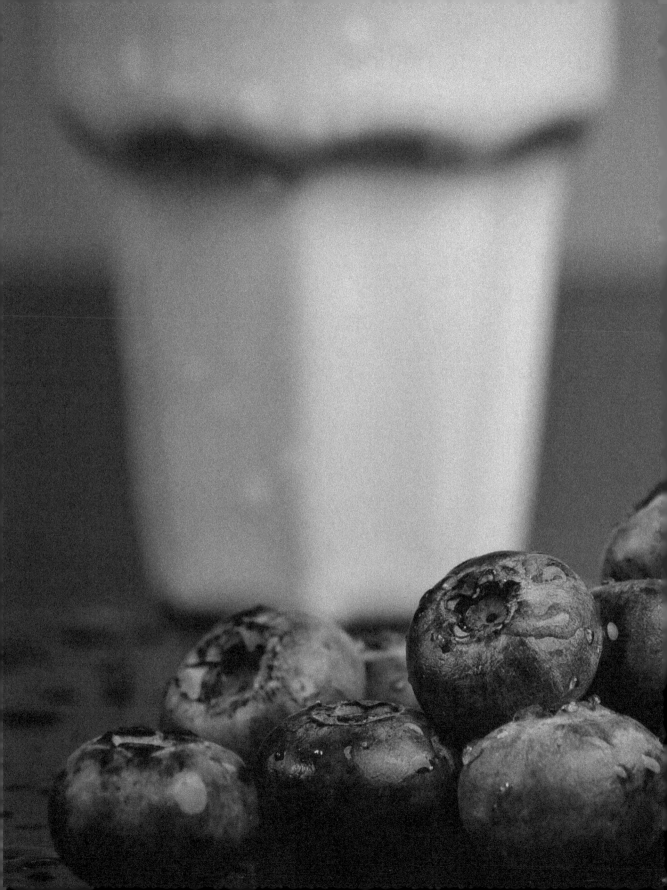

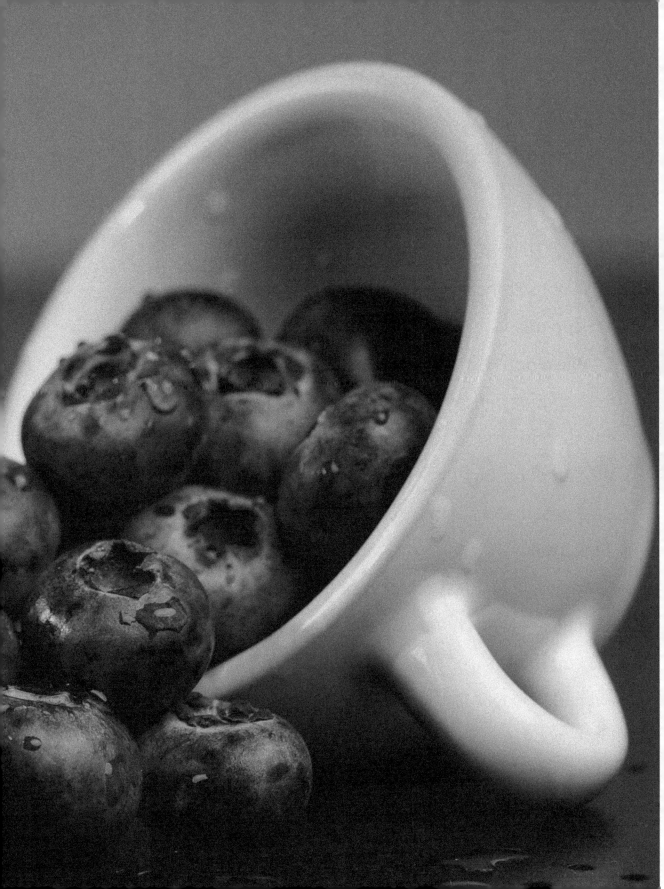

LENTIL AND RICE SALAD

Prep Time: 15 minutes | Cook Time: 20 minutes | Yield: 4 servings

Ingredients

1 1/4 cups French green lentils, rinsed, drained

1/3 cup fresh lime juice

2 tablespoons extra-virgin olive oil

4 teaspoons minced garlic

1 teaspoon ground cumin

3/4 teaspoon sugar

Kosher salt and freshly ground black pepper

2 cups steamed brown rice or brown basmati rice, cooled

1 tomato, halved, seeded, chopped

1/3 cup coarsely chopped fresh cilantro plus sprigs for garnish

1/3 cup thinly sliced red onion (from about 1/4 onion)

Avocado wedges (optional)

Lime wedges

DIRECTIONS

1. Place lentils in a saucepan and add water to cover by 3". Bring to a boil. Reduce heat to a simmer and cook, adding more water if needed to keep lentils covered, until lentils are tender, about 20 minutes. Drain; spread out lentils on a baking sheet and let cool.

2. Meanwhile, whisk lime juice, oil, garlic, cumin, and sugar in a small bowl to combine. Season dressing to taste with salt and pepper.

3. Combine cooled lentils, rice, tomato, chopped cilantro, and onion in a large bowl. Pour dressing over and gently mix to coat well; season to taste with more salt and pepper. Top with avocado, if using. Garnish with cilantro sprigs and lime wedges for squeezing over.

WALDORF SALAD

Prep Time: 15 minutes | Cook Time: - minutes | Yield: 4 servings

Ingredients

6 Tbsp mayonnaise (or plain yogurt)

1 Tbsp lemon juice

1/2 teaspoon salt

Pinch of freshly ground black pepper

2 sweet apples, cored and chopped

1 cup red seedless grapes, sliced in half (or 1/4 cup of raisins)

1 cup celery, thinly sliced

1 cup chopped, slightly toasted walnuts

Lettuce

DIRECTIONS

In a medium sized bowl, whisk together the mayonnaise (or yogurt), lemon juice, salt and pepper. Stir in the apple, celery, grapes, and walnuts. Serve on a bed of fresh lettuce.

TOASTED PITA TRIANGLES

Prep Time: 20 minutes | Cook Time: 20 minutes | Yield: 4 servings

Ingredients

6 whole pitas, split in half and cut into triangles

pan spray, or olive oil

2 teaspoons garlic salt

1/2 teaspoon freshly ground black pepper

DIRECTIONS

1. Split the pitas and cut into triangles.
2. Lay them on a shallow baking dish in a single layer inside up.
3. Lightly film the insides with olive oil, using a brush or spray. Sprinkle liberally with seasoning.
4. Bake until golden brown, about 8 minutes.
5. Remove from oven to cool. They will become crisp as they cool.

TURKEY BURGERS WITH TOMATO CORN SALSA

Prep Time: 5 minutes | Cook Time: 20 minutes | Yield: 4 servings

Ingredients

For the salsa:

12 cherry tomatoes, finely chopped

1/2 teaspoon kosher salt

1/2 cup cooked fresh corn or

thawed frozen corn kernels

1 tablespoon fresh lime juice

1 garlic clove, minced

1 tablespoon chopped fresh cilantro

2 teaspoons olive oil

Additional kosher salt and freshly ground

black pepper to taste.

For the burgers:

2 tablespoons vegetable oil

1 small onion, finely chopped

1/2 small red bell pepper, finely chopped

1 tablespoon store-bought or homemade Creole Spice Mix (recipe follows)

1 teaspoon kosher salt

Freshly ground black pepper to taste

DIRECTIONS

To make the salsa, toss the tomatoes with the salt and drain in a colander for 15 minutes. Combine the tomatoes, corn, lime juice, garlic, cilantro, and olive oil in a large bowl. Season with salt and pepper and toss well. To prepare the burgers, preheat the oven to 400°F. Heat 1 tablespoon of the oil in a small skillet over medium heat. Add the onion and red pepper and cook, until softened, about 5 minutes. Cool to room temperature.

Combine the onion, pepper, Creole spice mix, salt, and turkey in a large bowl. Season with pepper. Mix well and form into 4 patties. Heat the remaining tablespoon of oil in a large ovenproof grill pan or skillet over medium heat. Place the burgers in the skillet and cook until well browned, about 5 minutes per side. Transfer to the oven and cook until firm to the touch, about 6 minutes. Serve topped with the salsa.

Creole Spice Mix: Mix 4 teaspoons hot paprika, 1 tablespoon kosher salt, 1 tablespoon garlic powder, 1 1/2 teaspoons freshly ground black pepper, 1 1/2 teaspoons onion powder, 1 1/2 teaspoons cayenne pepper, 1 1/2 teaspoons dried oregano, 1 1/2 teaspoons dried thyme in a small bowl. Store in an airtight container. Makes about 1/2 cup.

CHICKEN TABBOULEH SALAD

Prep Time: 20 minutes | Cook Time: 50 minutes | Yield: 4 servings

Ingredients

Chicken:

2 tsp smoked paprika

1/2 tsp turmeric

2 tsp ground cumin

1/2 tsp cinnamon

2 tsp pepper or to taste

1 tsp salt or to taste

1/4 cup lemon juice

1/2 cup olive oil

1 tsp red pepper flakes

4 cloves garlic minced

1 lb chicken breasts boneless and skinless

1 large onion sliced

Tabbouleh Salad:

2 cups water

1 cup bulgur wheat uncooked

1/4 cup olive oil

1/4 cup lemon juice

3 cups tomatoes chopped small

1 English cucumber chopped small

1/4 cup green onions chopped

2 cups fresh parsley chopped

1/4 cup fresh mint chopped

1/4 tsp salt or to taste

1/4 tsp pepper or to taste

DIRECTIONS

For Chicken:

1. In a 8×8 baking dish add the smoked paprika, turmeric, cumin, cinnamon, pepper, salt, lemon juice, olive oil, red pepper flakes, garlic, and whisk well. Add the chicken, sliced onion and toss making sure the chicken is well coated in the marinade. Cover with plastic wrap or foil and refrigerate for at least an hour. The longer the meat marinates the more flavour you'll have.

2. Preheat the oven to 425 F degrees.

3. Bake uncovered until the chicken is browned and crisp on the edges, and cooked through. It should take about 40 to 45 minutes. If you want the chicken crispier on top, turn the broiler on to high and broil for 3 minutes until nice and crispy on the outside.

4. Let the chicken rest for 5 to 10 minutes before slicing

Tabbouleh Salad:

1. While the chicken is baking, prepare the tabbouleh salad. Add the water to a small pot and bring to boil. When the water is boiling add the bulgur and cover. Reduce heat to a simmer and

cook for about 5 minutes or until all the water is absorbed. Stir occasionally. Let the bulgur cool before adding to the salad.

2. Add the bulgur to a large bowl, then add the remaining ingredients. Toss well.

3. To assemble the salad, spread the tabbouleh salad over the bottom of a large shallow plate. Arrange with sliced chicken, sliced avocado, Kalamata olives and sprinkle some feta cheese over the top. Serve with hummus and pita bread.

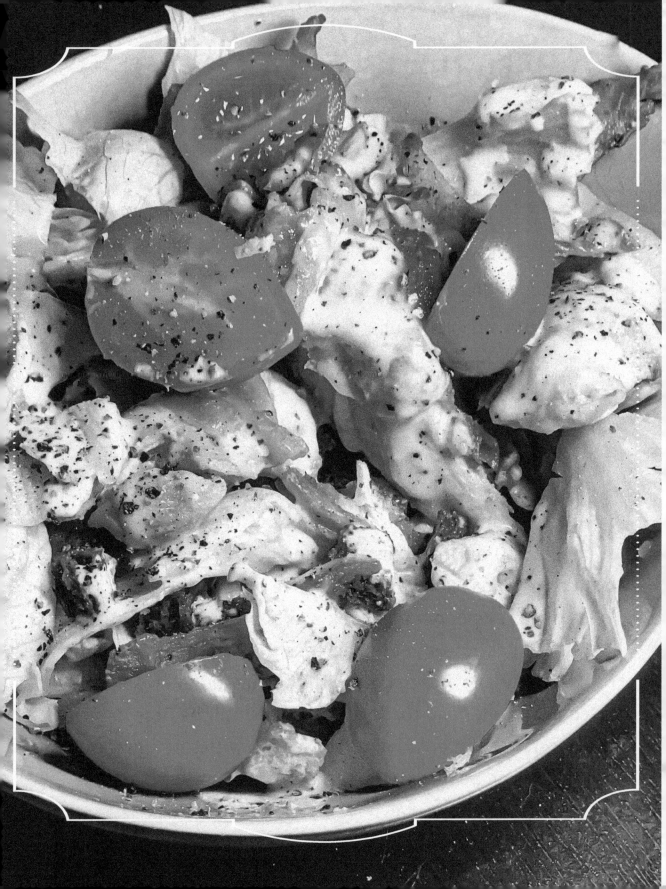

GARLICKY BROCCOLINI

Prep Time: 10 minutes | Cook Time: 15 minutes | Yield: 8 servings

Ingredients

Salt 2 pounds Broccolini (about 4 bunches)

1/4 cup extra-virgin olive oil

4 garlic cloves, thinly sliced

1 teaspoon crushed red pepper

DIRECTIONS

1. Bring a large pot of salted water to a boil. Add the Broccolini and cook until bright green and barely crisp-tender, about 5 minutes. Drain, reserving 1/2 cup of the cooking water.
2. In a very large skillet, heat the olive oil with the garlic and crushed red pepper and cook over moderate heat until fragrant, about 1 minute. Increase the heat to high, add the Broccolini and toss to coat with the oil. Add the reserved cooking water and toss occasionally, until the Broccolini is crisp-tender, about 2 minutes. Season with salt and transfer to a platter. Serve warm or at room temperature.

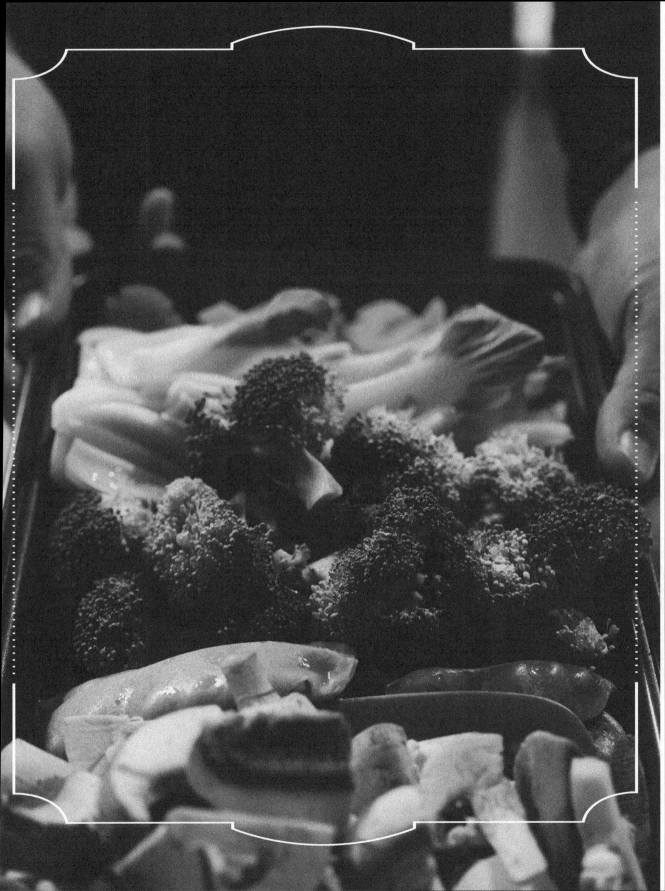

MIXED BERRY FRUIT SALAD

Prep Time: 15 minutes | Cook Time: 0 minutes | Yield: 2 servings

Ingredients

Strawberries

Blackberries

Blueberries

Fresh Mint

Lemon Juice or Lime Juice

DIRECTIONS

A simple fruit salad is the perfect side dish. Combine three types of fresh berries and create a mixed berry salad that everyone loves. It takes less than 15 minutes to put together and is great for serving for any time of the day. Make it ahead of time or just prior to serving. Either way, it's delicious, refreshing and flavorful.

In a bowl add the berries and lemon juice, mix well. Garnish with fresh mint leaves, as desired.

You can also use fresh raspberries in this salad but raspberries are softer so be careful not to crush them when mixing. The raspberries are best when serving immediately.

MANHATTAN CLAM CHOWDER

Prep Time: 10 minutes | Cook Time: 45 minutes | Yield: 6 servings

Ingredients

2 slices bacon (can sub with 2 more Tbsp extra virgin olive oil)

1 tablespoon extra virgin olive oil

2 carrots, peeled and sliced

2 celery stalks, chopped

1 onion, chopped

1 large garlic clove, minced

1/2 teaspoon dried thyme

1/4 teaspoon celery seed

2 bay leaves

12 ounces of tomato juice, strained tomatoes or crushed tomatoes

1 14-ounce can of clam broth

or juice*

2 10-ounce cans of baby clams, juice reserved*

1 pound waxy potatoes, peeled and cut into 2-inch chunks

A dozen or so live small clams, such as littlenecks or Manila clams

Salt and black pepper to taste

Tabasco or other hot sauce

If using fresh quahogs, scrub clean a dozen or more quahogs. Place clams in a small pot and add two cups of water. Bring water to a boil. Cover the pot and steam the clams until they completely open, about 10 to 20 minutes. Remove from heat. Remove clams from pot and set aside. Strain the clam steaming liquid through a fine mesh sieve or cheesecloth to catch any grit, reserving the liquid. Remove the clams from the shells, chop. Use chopped clams in place of canned. Use steaming liquid in place of clam broth.

DIRECTIONS

1. Cook the bacon: Slowly cook the bacon with the olive oil on medium heat until the bacon is crispy and its fat rendered. Remove, chop and set aside.
2. Cook the carrots, celery, onion, then garlic: Increase the heat to medium-high and sauté the carrots, celery and onion until soft and translucent, about 4-5 minutes. Do not brown the vegetables. Add the garlic and cook for another minute. Return chopped bacon to the pot.
3. Add the herbs, tomato juice, clam broth and the juice from the canned clams, mix well, then add the potatoes. Bring to a simmer, cover and simmer gently until the potatoes are done, about 30-40 minutes.
4. Add clams: When the potatoes are tender, add the canned clams

cover the pot and simmer until the live clams open up, about 5-10 minutes.

5. Add Tabasco, salt and black pepper to taste.
6. Place a clam in shell or two in each bowl for serving.

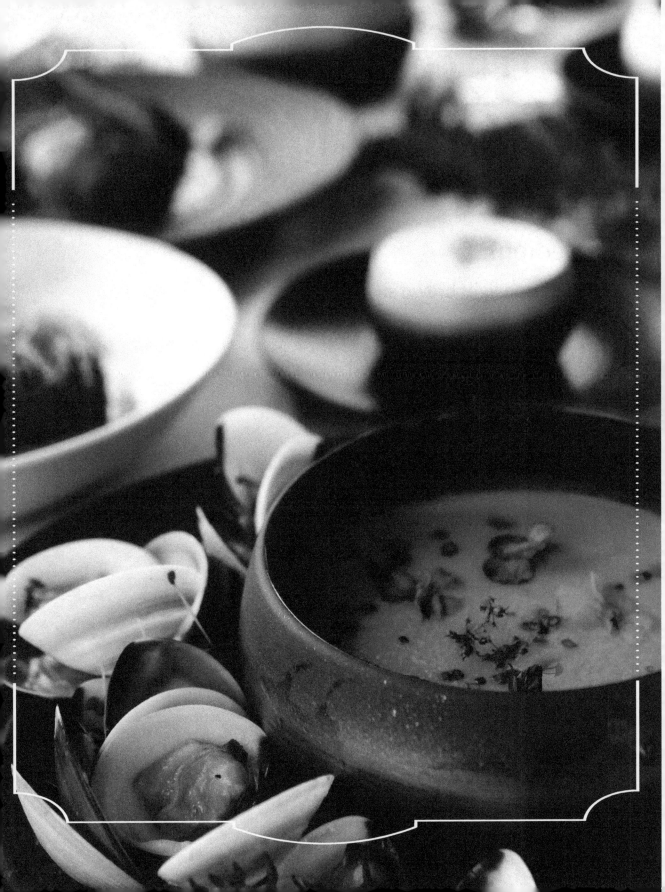

GRILLED CHICKEN WITH TOMATO-CUCUMBER SALAD

Prep Time: 25 minutes | Cook Time: 15 minutes | Yield: 4 servings

Ingredients

1 tablespoon light brown sugar

1 teaspoon smoked paprika

2 teapoons kosher salt, divided

1 teaspoon black pepper, divided

4 12-ounce chicken leg quarters

2 tablespoons olive oil, divided

2 pounds heirloom tomatoes, cut into ½-in.-thick wedges

1 English cucumber, thinly sliced

2 tabelspoons fresh lemon juice (from 1 lemon)

¼ cup fresh basil leaves

DIRECTIONS

1. Prepare a grill for indirect medium-high heat. Combine brown sugar, paprika, 1 teaspoon salt, and ½ teaspoon pepper. Brush chicken with 1 tablespoon oil; season with brown sugar mixture.

2. Place chicken, skin side down, over direct heat. Grill until lightly charred, 5 to 10 minutes. Flip and transfer to indirect heat. Cover and cook until a thermometer inserted in thickest part registers 165°F, 35 to 40 minutes.

3. Meanwhile, toss tomatoes with cucumber, lemon juice, and remaining 1 tablespoon oil, 1 teaspoon salt, and ½ teaspoon pepper. Top with basil and serve with chicken.

HEALTHY CARROT MUFFINS

Prep Time: 15 minutes | Cook Time: 13 minutes | Yield: 12 muffins

Ingredients

1 ¾ cups white whole wheat flour or regular whole wheat flour

1 ½ teaspoons baking powder

1 teaspoon ground cinnamon

½ teaspoon baking soda

½ teaspoon salt

½ teaspoon ground ginger

¼ teaspoon ground nutmeg

2 cups peeled and grated carrots* (from ¾ pound carrots—about 3 large or up to 6 small/medium)

½ cup roughly chopped walnuts

½ cup raisins (I like golden raisins), tossed in 1 teaspoon flour

⅓ cup melted coconut oil or extra-virgin olive oil

½ cup maple syrup or honey

2 eggs, preferably at room temperature

1 cup plain Greek yogurt

1 teaspoon vanilla extract

1 tablespoon turbinado sugar (also called raw sugar), for sprinkling on top

DIRECTIONS

1. Preheat oven to 425 degrees Fahrenheit. If necessary, grease all 12 cups on your muffin tin with butter or non-stick cooking spray.

2. In a large mixing bowl, combine the flour, baking powder, cinnamon, baking soda, salt, ginger and nutmeg. Blend well with a whisk. In a separate, small bowl, toss the raisins with 1 teaspoon flour so they don't stick together. Add the grated carrots, chopped walnuts and floured raisins to the other ingredients and stir to combine.

3. In a medium mixing bowl, combine the oil and maple syrup and beat together with a whisk. Add the eggs and beat well, then add the yogurt and vanilla and mix well. (If the coconut oil solidifies in contact with cold ingredients, gently warm the mixture in the microwave in 30 second bursts.)

4. Pour the wet ingredients into the dry and mix with a big spoon, just until combined (a few lumps are ok). Divide the batter evenly between the 12 muffin cups. Sprinkle the tops of the muffins with turbinado sugar. Bake muffins for 13 to 16 minutes, or until the muffins are golden on top and a toothpick inserted into a muffin comes out clean.

5. Place the muffin tin on a cooling rack to cool.

SICILIAN-STYLE CAULIFLOWER WITH WHOLE WHEAT PASTA

Prep Time: 15 minutes | Cook Time: 25 minutes | Yield: 6 servings

Ingredients

2 teaspoons kosher salt

¾ pound pasta, penne

¼ cup olive oil, extra-virgin

5 cups cauliflower florets (3/4-inch, about 1 to 1 1/4 pounds)

1 large shallots

2 cloves garlic smashed

¾ cup water

¼ cup white wine vinegar

2 teaspoons golden raisins

1 tablespoon honey

1 tablespoon capers

1 each thyme sprigs

1 each bay leaves

2 teaspoons fennel seeds

DIRECTIONS

1. Bring a large pot of water to a boil over high heat, then salt it generously.
2. Add the penne and cook, stirring occasionally, until al dente?o tender but not mushy.
3. Drain the pasta in a colander set in the sink.
4. Transfer to a large bowl.
5. Meanwhile, heat 2 tablespoons of the oil in a large skillet over medium-high heat.
6. Add the cauliflower, shallots, and garlic, and cook, stirring, until the cauliflower is well browned, about 8 minutes.
7. Reduce the heat to medium.
8. Add the remaining 2 tablespoons oil, 2 teaspoons salt, water, vinegar, raisins, honey, capers, thyme, bay leaf, fennel seeds, if using, and season with black pepper.
9. Bring to a simmer, cover, and cook until cauliflower is fork tender, about 7 to 8 minutes.
10. Remove from the heat and add the pine nuts and parsley.
11. Remove and discard the thyme and bay leaf.
12. Toss vegetables and pasta together along with the pecorino.
13. Drizzle with additional olive oil, if desired.
14. Serve immediately, passing more cheese at the table.

CHICKEN AND PASTA SOUP

Prep Time: 20 minutes | Cook Time: 30 minutes | Yield: 12 servings

Ingredients

2 tablespoons extra virgin olive oil

¾ cup finely chopped shallots about 2 large shallots

3 medium celery stalks diced

8 medium carrots peeled and diced

12 cups low sodium chicken broth

2 medium bay leaves

1 teaspoon finely chopped fresh rosemary and thyme each

1½ teaspoons kosher salt if you're using regular salt, start with a half teaspoon and add more, if needed.

¼ teaspoon freshly ground black pepper

1 cup Acini di pepe pasta You can also use pastina, orzo or Israeli couscous, also known as pearl pasta.

3-4 cups leftover turkey or chicken diced, rotisserie chicken works great

1 teaspoon finely chopped fresh rosemary (to finish)

DIRECTIONS

1. Heat olive oil over medium heat in a large Dutch oven or pot. Add chopped shallots and cook for 2 minutes, stirring frequently. Add celery and carrots and cook for another 3-4 minutes, stirring frequently.

2. Add the broth, bay leaves, fresh rosemary and thyme, salt and pepper. Bring soup to a boil then reduce to a steady simmer and cook, uncovered for 20 minutes.

3. Remove bay leaves and add the Acini di pepe pasta. Stir and return to a simmer. Cook for 8-10 more minutes, or until pasta is tender.

4. Add diced chicken (or turkey), rosemary and thyme. Stir well and remove from heat. Taste and add more salt and/ or pepper, as needed. Cover and allow soup to sit for 15 minutes before serving. This allows the flavors to meld.

LINGUINE WITH SHRIMP

Prep Time: 10 minutes | Cook Time: 25 minutes | Yield: 4 servings

Ingredients

1 lb. linguine

1 tbsp. extra-virgin olive oil

1 lb. shrimp, peeled and deveined

Kosher salt

Freshly ground black pepper

4 tbsp. butter

3 cloves garlic, minced

1/2 tsp. crushed red pepper flakes, plus more for garnish

2 1/2 c. grape tomatoes, halved

1/4 c. white wine

1 c. heavy cream

Juice of 1 lemon

5 oz. baby kale (about 6 c.)

1/2 c. freshly grated Parmesan, plus more for garnish

DIRECTIONS

1. In a large pot of salted boiling water, cook linguine according to the package directions until al dente. Drain, reserving ½ cup pasta water, and return to pot.

2. In a large skillet over medium heat, heat oil. Add shrimp and season with salt and pepper. Cook until shrimp is pink and cooked through, 4 minutes. Remove from skillet and reserve on a plate.

3. Add butter to skillet then add garlic and red pepper flakes and cook until fragrant, 1 minute. Add tomatoes to skillet and cook until beginning to soften, 3 minutes. Season with salt and pepper. Add wine and cook until mostly reduced, 5 minutes.

4. Add heavy cream, lemon juice, and Parmesan. Let simmer until sauce is thickened, 5 minutes. Add pasta, shrimp, and kale and toss to coat. If sauce is too thick, add additional pasta water.

MANGO STRAWBERRY SNOW CONES

Prep Time: 10 minutes | Cook Time: - minutes | Yield: 4 servings

Ingredients

ice

2 mangoes peeled and chopped

1 pint strawberries hulled and sliced

1 lime juiced plus wedges for garnish

DIRECTIONS

1. Fill a food processor with ice.
2. Process until the ice is very fine, like snow.
3. Add the mangoes and strawberries and pulse to blend.
4. Pile the crushed ice into dessert glasses or dishes and squeeze over the lime juice.
5. Garnish with lime wedges; serve immediately.

PEACH FRENCH TOAST

Prep Time: 20 minutes | Cook Time: 45 minutes | Yield: 6 servings

Ingredients

1 cup packed brown sugar

1/2 cup butter, cubed

2 tablespoons water

1 can (29 ounces) sliced peaches, drained

12 slices day-old French bread (3/4 inch thick)

5 large eggs

1-1/2 cups whole milk

1 tablespoon vanilla extract

Ground cinnamon

DIRECTIONS

1. In a small saucepan, bring the brown sugar, butter and water to a boil. Reduce heat; simmer for 10 minutes, stirring frequently. Pour into a greased 13x9-in. baking dish; top with peaches. Arrange bread over peaches.

2. In a large bowl, whisk the eggs, milk and vanilla; slowly pour over bread. Cover and refrigerate for 8 hours or overnight.

3. Preheat oven to 350°. Remove dish from the refrigerator 30 minutes before baking; sprinkle with cinnamon. Cover and bake 20 minutes. Uncover; bake until a knife inserted in the center of French toast comes out clean, 25-30 minutes longer. Serve with a spoon.

GREEK SALAD WITH OREGANO MARINATED CHICKEN

Prep Time: 10 minutes | Cook Time: 5 minutes | Yield: 4 servings

Ingredients

Vinaigrette:

3 tablespoons red wine vinegar

3 tablespoons lemon juice

2 teaspoons Dijon mustard

1 teaspoon minced garlic

1 teaspoon dried oregano leaves

1/4 cup plain nonfat yogurt

2 tablespoons olive oil

pinch sugar

Salad:

3 tablespoons lemon juice

1 tablespoon olive oil

1 teaspoon dried oregano leaves

-- Salt and pepper

1 1/2pounds boneless, skinless chicken breasts

4 cups mixed greens

1 cup peeled, cubed, cucumber chunks

1 cup cherry or grape tomatoes, halved

1/2 cup coarsely chopped red onion

1/3 cup pittted coarsely chopped kalamata olives

1/4 cup crumbled reduced-fat feta cheese

3 tablespoons pine nuts, toasted

DIRECTIONS

1. To prepare the vinaigrette: In small bowl, whisk together vinegar, lemon juice, mustard, garlic, and oregano. Stir in yogurt and then add olive oil, mixing well. Add sugar, if desired. Makes about 2/3 cup dressing

2. To prepare the salad: In plastic ziptop bag or glass container, combine lemon juice, olive oil, oregano, and salt and pepper. Add chicken breasts, thoroughly coating with mixture.

3. Marinate in refrigerator atleast 30 minutes and up to 4 hours. Discard marinade and cook chicken on nonstick grill pan or skillet coated with nonstick cooking spray 4 to 5 minutes on each side or until done. Remove from pan and slice. Set chicken aside.

4. In large bowl, combine greens, cucumber, tomatoes, onion, olives and cheese. Toss salad with vinaigrette and top with chicken strips.

CRAB CAKES

Prep Time: 10 minutes | Cook Time: 10 minutes | Yield: 4 servings

Ingredients

1/3 c. mayonnaise

1 large egg, beaten

2 tbsp. Dijon mustard

2 tsp. Worcestershire sauce

1/2 tsp. hot sauce

Kosher salt

Freshly ground black pepper

1 lb. jumbo lump crabmeat, picked over for shells

3/4 c. panko bread crumbs (or saltines)

2 tbsp. Freshly Chopped Parsley

Canola oil, for frying

Lemon wedges, for serving

Tartar sauce, for serving

DIRECTIONS

1. In a small bowl, whisk together mayo, egg, Dijon mustard, Worcestershire, and hot sauce, and season with salt and pepper.
2. In a medium bowl, stir together crabmeat, panko, and parsley. Fold in mayo mixture, then form into 8 patties.
3. In a large skillet over medium-high heat, coat pan with oil and heat until shimmering. Add crab cakes and cook, in batches, until golden and crispy, 3 to 5 minutes per side.
4. Serve wlth lemon and tartar sauce

POACHED SALMON WITH LEMON MINT TZATZIKI SAUCE

Prep Time: 3 hours | Cook Time: 8 minutes | Yield: 4 servings

Ingredients

2 cups dry white wine

2 cups water

2 bay leaves

2 sprigs flat-leaf parsley

2 lemons, unpeeled, sliced

1 (2 lb) salmon fillet with skin

1 scallion, top only, thinly sliced

1 cup Lemon Mint Tzatziki Sauce (recipe below)

Mint Tzatziki Sauce :

1 cucumber

1 cup plain, nonfat yogurt, drained

1 tsp olive oil

2 tsp lemon juice

1/2 tsp minced garlic

1/4 tsp lemon zest

1 tbsp chopped mint

DIRECTIONS

1. Put the wine, water, bay leaves, parsley, and 1 sliced lemon into a large, deep skillet; bring to a simmer.
2. Add salmon, skin-side down. (Add more water, if necessary, to cover the salmon.) Cover skillet and simmer over low heat until the fish is just cooked through, about 8 minutes.
3. Transfer fish to a plate, cover, and refrigerate until completely chilled, about 3 hours.
4. Peel skin from fillet and scrape away any brown flesh.
5. Serve fish over sautéed baby spinach and top with the scallion, remaining lemon slices, and Lemon Mint Tzatziki Sauce. Pair with a cup of cooked orzo.

- **To make the sauce:**
- Peel, seed, and grate the cucumber. Drain it well. In a medium bowl, stir together the yogurt and olive oil. Add the cucumber, lemon juice, garlic, zest, and mint leaves; mix well. Season with salt and pepper to taste, and serve. For an even thicker sauce, line a strainer with a paper towel and put the strainer over a bowl. Put the yogurt in the strainer and place it in the refrigerator to drain and thicken for 3 hours.

TAHINI EDAMAME BURGER

Prep Time: 20 minutes | Cook Time: 20 minutes | Yield: - servings

Ingredients

1 Tbsp. olive oil

1 large yellow onion, rough chopped

6 garlic cloves, whole

1 small sweet potato, rough chopped

2 cups fresh edamame, shelled and steamed in the microwave

6 cups packed mixed greens (spinach, baby kale), torn

1 heaping cup rolled oats

1/4 cup liquid amino acids or soy sauce

1/4 cup tahini

3 Tbsp. nutritional yeast

2 tsp. ground cumin

1 tsp. fresh chili paste

DIRECTIONS

1. Heat the olive oil in a large rimmed frying pan over medium. In a food processor, pulse the onion and garlic until finely diced. Add the mixture to the pan and saute for about 5 minutes.

2. Meanwhile, pulse the sweet potato in the food processor until finely diced. Add to the frying pan.

3. Pulse the shelled edamame in the processor until finely diced. Add to the frying pan. Saute the vegetable mixture for about 10-15 minutes, over medium-high heat, until all the water is evaporated and the sweet potato is tender. You want the mixture to start sticking to the bottom.

4. Now, pulse the oats in the food processor until roughly ground. Add to the vegetable mixture and stir to combine.

5. Whisk together the remaining ingredients in a small bowl until smooth. Stir into the vegetable mixture until very well combined and remove from heat.

6. Heat a cast iron skillet with a dash of olive oil over medium-high heat. Form 1/4 cup of the burger mixture into a patty and brown on each side for a couple minutes. Repeat with remaining burger mixture.

7. Serve hot.

APPLE MUFFINS

Prep Time: 20 minutes | Cook Time: 20 minutes | Yield: - servings

Ingredients

1 ¾ cups white whole wheat flour or regular whole wheat flour

1 ½ teaspoons baking powder

1 teaspoon ground cinnamon

½ teaspoon baking soda

½ teaspoon salt

1 cup grated apple

1 cup apple diced into ¼" cubes

⅓ cup melted coconut oil or extra-virgin olive oil

½ cup maple syrup or honey*

2 eggs, preferably at room temperature

½ cup plain Greek yogurt (I used full-fat but any variety should do)

½ cup applesauce

1 teaspoon vanilla extract

1 tablespoon turbinado sugar (also called raw sugar), for sprinkling on top

DIRECTIONS

1. Preheat oven to 425 degrees Fahrenheit. If necessary, grease all 12 cups on your muffin tin with butter or non-stick cooking spray

2. In a large mixing bowl, combine the flour, baking powder, cinnamon, baking soda and salt. Blend well with a whisk. Add the grated apple (if it is dripping wet, gently squeeze it over the sink to release some extra moisture) and chopped apple. Stir to combine.

3. In a medium mixing bowl, combine the oil and maple syrup and beat together with a whisk. Add the eggs and beat well, then add the yogurt, applesauce and vanilla and mix well. (If the coconut oil solidifies in contact with cold ingredients, gently warm the mixture in the microwave in 30 second bursts.)

4. Pour the wet ingredients into the dry and mix with a big spoon, just until combined (a few lumps are ok). The batter will be thick, but don't worry! Divide the batter evenly between the 12 muffin cups. Sprinkle the tops of the muffins with turbinado sugar. Bake muffins for 13 to 16 minutes, or until the muffins are golden on top and a toothpick inserted into a muffin comes out clean.

5. Place the muffin tin on a cooling rack to cool.

BAKED MAHI MAHI WITH WINE AND HERBS

Prep Time: 20 minutes | Cook Time: 20 minutes | Yield: 4 servings

Ingredients

4 sprigs Fresh Thyme

8 sprigs Fresh Parsley

3 Bay Leaves, preferably fresh

8 cloves Garlic, smashed

4 (6-ounce) skinless Mahi Mahi fillets

Kosher salt and freshly ground black pepper

3/4 c dry White Wine – Sauvignon Blanc

4 T Extra-Virgin Olive Oil

2 t freshly squeezed Lemon Juice, Meyer's Lemon

12 Cherry or Pear Red and Yellow tomatoes, for garnish

DIRECTIONS

1. Preheat oven to 450 degrees F.
2. Make a bed of herbs in a medium gratin dish or baking dish with the thyme, 4 of the parsley sprigs, and the bay leaves. Scatter the garlic on top. Season both sides of the fish with salt and pepper and place on top of the herbs. Add the Sauvignon Blanc and drizzle 2 tablespoons of the oil over the fish. Cover loosely with foil and bake until the fish is opaque, about 15 to 20 minutes, depending on how thick the fillets are.
3. Carefully pour the pan juices into a small saucepan and set the fish aside. Reserve the garlic and 4 thyme sprigs. Bring the sauce to a boil over high heat and cook until reduced by half, about 5 minutes. Whisk in the remaining 2 tablespoons olive oil and the lemon juice. Season with salt and pepper. Set aside.
4. Divide fish among 4 serving plates. Pour sauce over fish and garnish with the 4 remaining parsley sprigs, the reserved garlic and thyme, and tomatoes

MINESTRONE SOUP WITH PASTA AND BEANS

Prep Time: 10 minutes | Cook Time: 20 minutes | Yield: 8 servings

Ingredients

1 cup ditalini pasta , regular, whole wheat or gluten-free

Salt and ground black pepper , to taste

3 cloves garlic , minced

1 onion , diced

3 carrots , peeled and diced

2 stalks celery , diced

3 cups vegetable broth

15 oz Kidney beans , drained and rinsed well

15 oz cannellini beans , drained and rinsed well

15 oz tomato sauce

15 oz tomatoes, diced

1 1/4 cups zucchini ,and/or Yellow summer squash

1 tablespoon dried Italian Seasoning Spice Blend

DIRECTIONS

1. In a large pot of boiling salted water, cook pasta according to package instructions; drain well and set aside.
2. Heat 1 tablespoon olive oil in a large stockpot or Dutch oven over medium heat.
3. Stir in garlic, onion, carrots and celery. Cook, stirring occasionally, until tender, about 3-4 minutes.
4. Whisk in vegetable broth, tomato sauce, diced tomatoes, Italian Seasoning Spice blend, and Italian sausage; season with salt and pepper, to taste. Bring to a boil; reduce heat to a simmer. Cover the pot with a tight-fitting lid and cook until vegetables are tender, about 10-15 minutes.
5. Stir in the beans, zucchini, and summer squash until just heated through - about 3 minutes.
6. If serving the full soup with no anticipated leftovers, add the pasta to the soup and stir to combine. Otherwise, I add mine to the bowls at serving. Pasta

CRISPY CHICKEN TENDERS

Prep Time: 40 minutes | Cook Time: 20 minutes | Yield: 16 servings

Ingredients

4 chicken breasts boneless skinless

1 cup buttermilk

1 teaspoon hot sauce

2 large eggs beaten

2 cups flour

2 1/2 teaspoons salt

3/4 teaspoon pepper

1/8 teaspoon paprika

1/8 teaspoon garlic powder

1/8 teaspoon baking powder

canola oil for frying

DIRECTIONS

1. Cut the chicken breasts into four tenders each and soak them in a bowl with the buttermilk and hot sauce for 30 minutes.
2. Add the eggs to one bowl and the flour and spices to a second bowl.
3. Dip each piece of chicken from the buttermilk bowl to the flour mixture.
4. Dip it into the eggs then back into the flour mixture.
5. Shake excess flour gently off and put the chicken onto a baking sheet.
6. Repeat with all the pieces.
7. Heat the oil (three inches deep) in a dutch oven on medium high heat to 350 degrees.
8. Fry the chicken in small batches for 5-7 minutes or until golden brown.

SLOW-ROASTED SALMON WITH CUCUMBER DILL SALAD

Prep Time: 40 minutes | Cook Time: 20 minutes | Yield: 16 servings

Ingredients

The salmon:

4 (6-oz) salmon fillets, skin on

1 tablespoon extra virgin olive oil

kosher salt

freshly ground black pepper

For The Cucumber-Dill Salad

1 English cucumber (also called hothouse cucumber)

1/3 cup finely sliced red onion, from one small red onion

1/2 teaspoon salt

1/4 cup plus 2 tablespoons sour cream

3 tablespoons mayonnaise, best quality such as Hellmann's

or Duke's

2 tablespoons white wine vinegar

1/4 cup chopped fresh dill

1 clove garlic, minced

1/2 teaspoon sugar

freshly ground black pepper, to taste

DIRECTIONS

1. Cut the cucumber in half and then slice each half down the middle lengthwise. Use the tip of a teaspoon to scoop out the center seeds. Cut each half into thin slices and place in a colander along with the red onion slices. Toss with salt and let sit in the sink for at least 30 minutes, until the water drains out.

2. In the meantime, make the dressing: combine the sour cream, mayonnaise, white wine vinegar, dill, garlic, sugar and black pepper in a medium bowl and mix well.

3. When the cucumbers and onions are ready, release any excess water by tapping the colander on the base of the sink, then use a large wad of paper towels to pat the vegetables dry. Add to the dressing and toss well. Cover and chill until ready to serve.

4. Preheat the grill to medium-high heat. Clean the grill rack, then brush lightly with oil. Close the lid and let return to temperature. Rub the salmon with olive oil and season generously with kosher salt (about 3/4 teaspoon) and pepper. Place the fillets skin side down and grill until golden brown and slightly charred, 4-5 minutes (resist the urge to peek or flip early; when fillets are nicely seared on the first side, they should release easily). Flip the fillets over and continue

grilling until done, 2-3 minutes. Let cool slightly, remove the skin if desired, and serve with the cold cucumber-dill salad piled over top or alongside.

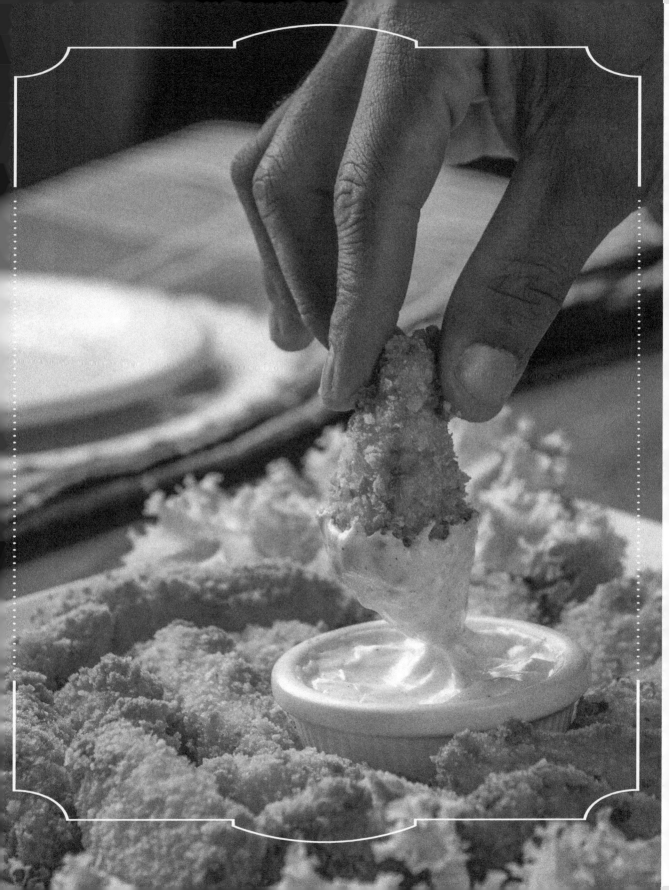

THAI SHRIMP STIR-FRY WITH TOMATOES AND BASIL

Prep Time: 15 minutes | Cook Time: 15 minutes | Yield: 3 servings

Ingredients

500 g large shrimp, peeled and deveined

1 medium yellow capsicum / bell pepper, sliced

1 small red onion, sliced

handful of basil leaves

1 punnet cherry tomatoes, halved

juice from 1 lime

2 tbsp soy sauce

2 tbsp water

1 tbsp brown sugar

1 tbsp fish sauce

1 tsp red chilli flakes

3 cloves garlic, minced

1 tbsp grated ginger

peanut oil

DIRECTIONS

1. In a small bowl mix and combine soy sauce, water, sugar and fish sauce.
2. In a wok heat oil. Once oil is hot sauté garlic, ginger, and chilli flakes until really fragrant.
3. Bring heat to really high then add the shrimps, stir fry until shrimps turn pink, roughly around 60 to 90 seconds. Remove everything from the wok place it in a plate then set it aside.
4. Back to your wok, add more oil if needed then stir fry onions and pepper, cook for 2 minutes. Add the shrimps back then pour the sauce mixture you made on step 1, bring to a boil while stir frying to distribute the sauce evenly.
5. Add the tomatoes and stir fry for 30 seconds.
6. Add the basil and lime juice then stir fry for 15 more seconds. Remove from wok then place in a serving platter then serve.

SNAPPER WITH GRAPE TOMATOES AND MUSHROOMS

Prep Time: 15 minutes | Cook Time: 15 minutes | Yield: 6 servings

Ingredients

6 red snapper fillets (about 8 oz. each)

1 container grape or cherry tomatoes (about 2 cups)

½ lb. mushrooms, coarsely chopped (about 2½ cups)

6 to 8 cloves garlic, peeled and sliced

1 Tablespoon dried or fresh thyme

Salt and freshly ground black pepper

2 Tablespoons chopped fresh basil, for garnish

Marinade:

¼ cup balsamic vinegar

2 Tablespoons olive oil

1 to 2 Tablespoons honey or maple syrup

1 Tablespoon lemon juice (preferably fresh)

DIRECTIONS

1. Line a large baking tray with foil and spray with cooking spray.
2. Arrange the fillets in a single layer on the prepared baking sheet.
3. Scatter the tomatoes, mushrooms, and garlic around the fish. Season with thyme, salt, and pepper to taste.
4. In a measuring cup, combine the vinegar, oil, honey, and lemon juice; mix well. Drizzle the mixture over the fish and vegetables until all are well coated. Marinate for 30 to 60 minutes.
5. Preheat the oven to 425°F. Bake the fish and vegetables, uncovered, for 12 to 15 minutes.
6. The fish is done when it just flakes when gently pressed with a fork.
7. Garnish with basil and serve immediately.

CHUNKY GUACAMOLE

Prep Time: 10 minutes | Cook Time: 15 minutes | Yield: 6 servings

Ingredients

3 large ripe avocados, peeled, pitted, and diced

1 large jalapeño, stemmed, seeded and finely-diced

half a medium red onion, peeled and diced

juice of 1 lime (about 2 Tablespoons)

1 cup diced tomatoes (such as cherry, grape, or roma tomatoes)

2/3 cup chopped fresh cilantro, loosely packed

1/2 teaspoon kosher salt, or more to taste

1/4 teaspoon ground cumin

DIRECTIONS

1. Add the avocadoes, jalapeno, red onion, lime juice, tomatoes, and cilantro to a large bowl. Sprinkle evenly with salt and cumin.
2. Using two spoons, toss the guacamole until it is evenly combined. Taste and season with extra salt if needed. (I usually like mine more salty.)
3. Serve immediately with chips for dipping.

CHOPPED NICOISE SALAD

Prep Time: 20 minutes | Cook Time: 12 minutes | Yield: 4 servings

Ingredients

2 large (free-range organic) eggs

12 oz / 340 gr red potatoes, peeled and cut into small dices

8 oz / 220 gr green beans

2 medium tomatoes, diced

4 tablespoons black olives, cut into slivers

5 oz / 140 gr herb salad mix or sliced romaine lettuce

2 tablespoons capers, drained

2 (5 oz / 140 gr) cans tuna in water, drained (I used Wild Planet wild albacore tuna)

2 tablespoons capers, drained

1 tablespoon chopped anchovies fillets (optional)

4 tablespoons olive oil

2 tablespoons vinegar

Fine grain sea salt

DIRECTIONS

1. Put the eggs in medium saucepan and cover with cold water by a ½-inch. Bring to a gently boil over medium-high heat. When the eggs start rattling against the bottom of the pan, turn off the heat, cover with a lid, and let sit for 12 minutes. Remove and run under cool water. Peel the eggs, roughly chop them, and put in the refrigerator.

2. In the meantime, bring a pot of water to a boil. Add diced potatoes and cook for about 10 minutes (you want the potatoes to retain a bit of crunch). Fish them out of the water with a slotted spoon, drain and let cool.

3. Add the green beans to water and cook for about 5 to 7 minutes. Drain and rinse with cold water. Transfer to a cutting board, chop them, and set aside.

4. Shake olive oil, vinegar, and salt in a tightly-lidded container or whisk together in a small bowl. Set aside.

5. To serve, combine in a large salad bowl (or in 4 individual bowls), herb salad mix, eggs, tomatoes, green beans, potatoes, black olives, capers, tuna, and anchovies (if using). Stir in vinaigrette.

6. Serve immediately.

CHICKEN CACCIATORE

Prep Time: 10 minutes | Cook Time: 40 minutes | Yield: 4 servings

Ingredients

3 tablespoons olive oil, divided

6 bone-in skinless chicken thighs

Salt and pepper, to season

1 medium onion, diced

2 tablespoons minced garlic, (or 6 cloves)

1 small yellow bell pepper (capsicum), diced

1 small red bell pepper (capsicum), diced

1 large carrot, peeled and sliced

10 oz (300g) mushrooms, sliced

1/2 cup pitted black olives

8 sprigs thyme

2 tablespoons each freshly chopped parsley and basil plus more to garnish

1 teaspoon dried oregano

150 ml red wine

28 oz (820g) crushed tomatoes

2 tablespoons tomato paste

7 oz (200g) Roma tomatoes, halved

1/2 teaspoon red pepper flakes

DIRECTIONS

1. Season chicken with salt and pepper.
2. Heat 2 tablespoons oil in a heavy cast iron skillet. Sear chicken on both sides until golden, about 3-4 minutes each side. Remove from skillet and set aside.
3. Add remaining oil to the pan. Sauté the onion until transparent, about 3-4 minutes. Add in garlic and cook until fragrant, about 30 seconds. Add the peppers, carrot, mushrooms and herbs; cook for 5 minutes until vegetables begin to soften.
4. Pour in the wine, scraping up browned bits from the bottom of the skillet. Cook until wine is reduced, about 2 minutes.
5. Add crushed tomatoes, tomato paste, Roma tomatoes and chill flakes. Season with salt and pepper to your tastes. Return chicken pieces to the skillet and continue to cook over stove top OR in the oven following the instructions below.

FOR STOVE TOP:

Mix all of the ingredients together; cover with lid, reduce heat to low and allow to simmer (while stirring occasionally) for 40 minutes or until the meat is falling off the bone. Add in the olives, allow to simmer for a further 10 minutes. Garnish with parsley and serve immediately.

FOR THE OVEN:

Transfer the covered skillet to a preheated oven at 375°F (190°C) and cook for 50 minutes. Remove the lid, add in the olives and cook for an additional 20 minutes until the chicken is tender and falling off the bone, and the sauce has reduced.

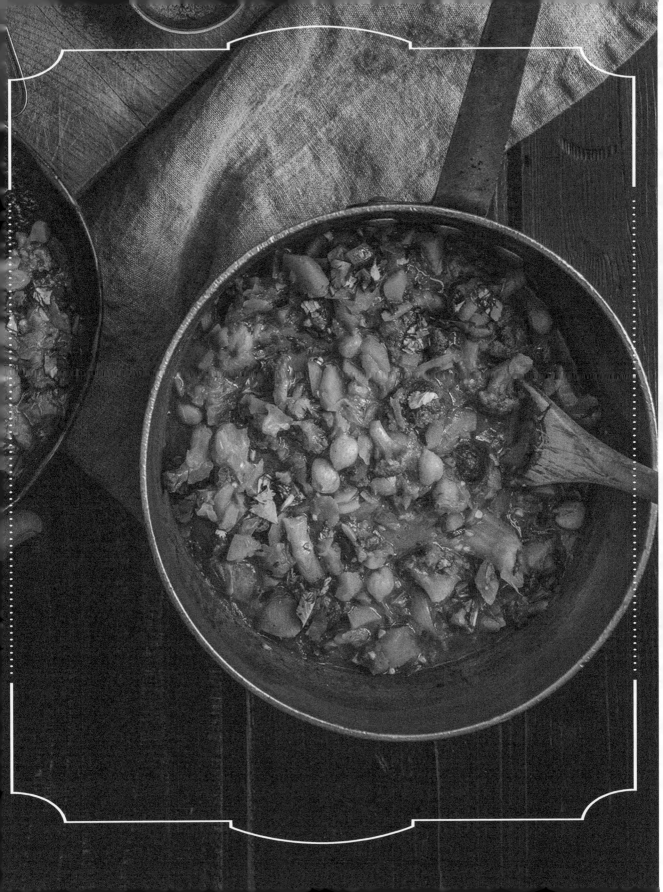

HOT CHOCOLATE

Prep Time: 10 minutes | Cook Time: 5 minutes | Yield: 1 servings

Ingredients

Unsweetened Cocoa Powder- 2 tablespoons per serving.

Sugar Alternative- 1 1/2 tablespoons equivalent to sugar.

Unsweetened almond milk or skim milk- 1 cup per serving.

You could use water instead but, don't expect the best tasting cocoa ever.

Vanilla Extract- 1/4 teaspoon per serving.

Salt- 1/4 teaspoon, can omit if avoiding salt.

Optional- Yay- Sugar Free Marshmallows

DIRECTIONS

1. In a sauce pan over medium heat, whisk together the cocoa powder, sugar alternative, and milk (or alternative).
2. When your cocoa is well blended and warm, remove from heat and whisk in the vanilla extract.
3. Serve with your optional sugar free marshmallow. Sometimes, I will use a bit of whipped cream.

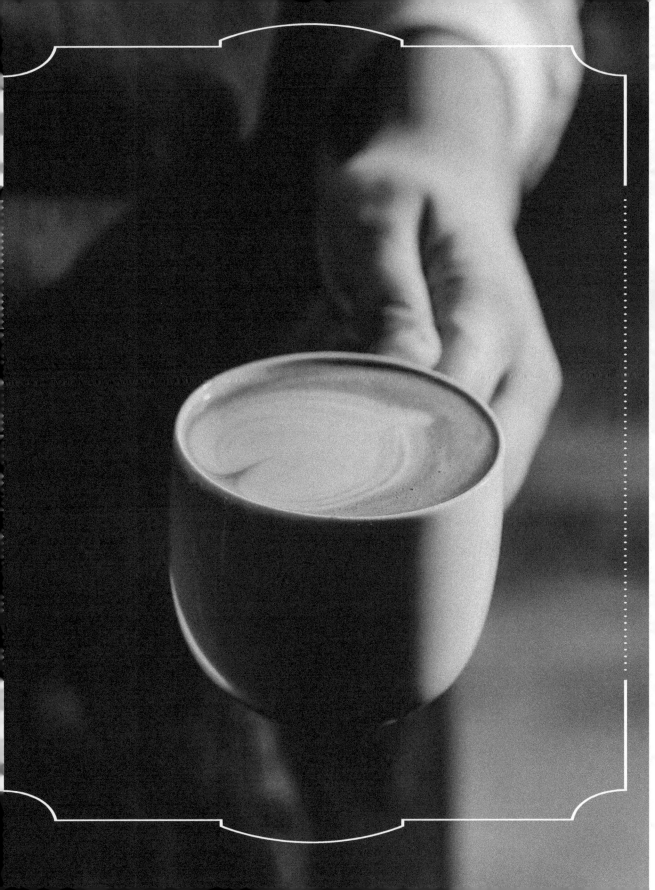

CHICKPEA AND SPINACH SALAD WITH CUMIN DRESSING

Prep Time: 15 minutes | Cook Time: 40 minutes | Yield: 4 servings

Ingredients

1 (15.5 ounce) can chickpeas, drained & rinsed

2 tablespoons chopped fresh flat-leaf parsley

1/4 cup diced red onion

2 tablespoons olive oil

2 tablespoons fresh lemon juice

1/4 teaspoon finely grated lemon zest

3/4 teaspoon ground cumin

pinch of cayenne pepper

salt & freshly ground black pepper to taste

3 tablespoons plain nonfat yogurt

1 tablespoon fresh squeezed orange juice

1/4 teaspoon finely grated orange zest

1/4 teaspoon honey

4 cups baby spinach leaves (packed)

1 tablespoon coarsely chopped fresh mint

DIRECTIONS

1. In a medium bowl, combine chickpeas, parsley and onion.
2. In a small bowl, whisk together the oil, lemon juice and zest, cumin, cayenne, salt and black pepper. Pour the dressing over the chickpea mixture and toss to coat evenly.
3. In another small bowl, stir together the yogurt, orange juice and zest, and honey.
4. Serve the chickpea salad over a bed of spinach leaves. Top with yogurt sauce and garnish with the mint.

SAN FRANCISCO CIOPPINO

Prep Time: 15 minutes | Cook Time: 50 minutes | Yield: 4 servings

Ingredients

1/2 cup butter

1 onion, chopped

1 fennel bulb, thinly sliced

4 cloves garlic, minced

1/2 bunch fresh parsley, chopped

1 tablespoon dried basil

1 teaspoon kosher salt

1/2 teaspoon dried thyme

1/2 teaspoon dried oregano

1/2 teaspoon crushed red pepper flakes

1 1/2 cups white wine (optional - can replace with additional fish or chicken stock)

1 (28 ounce) can crushed tomatoes

1 (14.5 ounce) can diced tomatoes

5 cups fish or seafood stock*

2 bay leaves

1 pound small clams

1 pound mussels, scrubbed and debearded

2 pounds crab (I used 1 whole cooked Dungeness crab, with its legs removed from its body)

1 pound uncooked large shrimp, peeled and deveined

1 pound bay scallops

1/2 pound cod fillet, cut into large chunks (or other firm-fleshed fish like halibut or salmon)

Fresh basil and parsley, chopped, for garnish

DIRECTIONS

1. Melt the butter over medium heat in a large stock pot, then add the onion, fennel, garlic, parsley, sauteing until the onions are soft, about 10 minutes. Add the garlic, basil, salt, thyme, oregano, and red pepper flakes and saute 2 minutes longer.
2. Add the white wine, crushed and diced tomatoes, fish stock, and bay leaves, then cover and reduce the heat to medium-low. Simmer for 30 minutes so the flavors can blend. While the meat simmers, prepare the crab by removing the crab legs from the body (if not already done for you) and using a nutcracker to crack the shells (leave the meat in the shell) so that the meat can be easily removed once the cioppino is served.
3. Increase the heat to medium and add the clams and mussels to the broth and cook for 5 minutes until they start to open. Then add the crab legs and cook for another minute, followed by the shrimp and scallops. Finally, lay the chunks of cod on top of the broth and cover and cook for 3-5 minutes until the mussels and clams are open, the shrimp curl and the scallops are just firm.
4. Ladle the cioppino into large bowls garnish with chopped fresh parsley and basil.

APPLEGURT

Prep Time: 3 minutes | Cook Time: - minutes | Yield: 1 servings

Ingredients

1/2 cup plain organic yogurt

1/2 cup unsweetened applesauce

1 tablespoon honey

1/2 cup granola or whole grain cereal

DIRECTIONS

Mix together yogurt, applesauce and honey. Chill for 20 minutes. Top with granola.

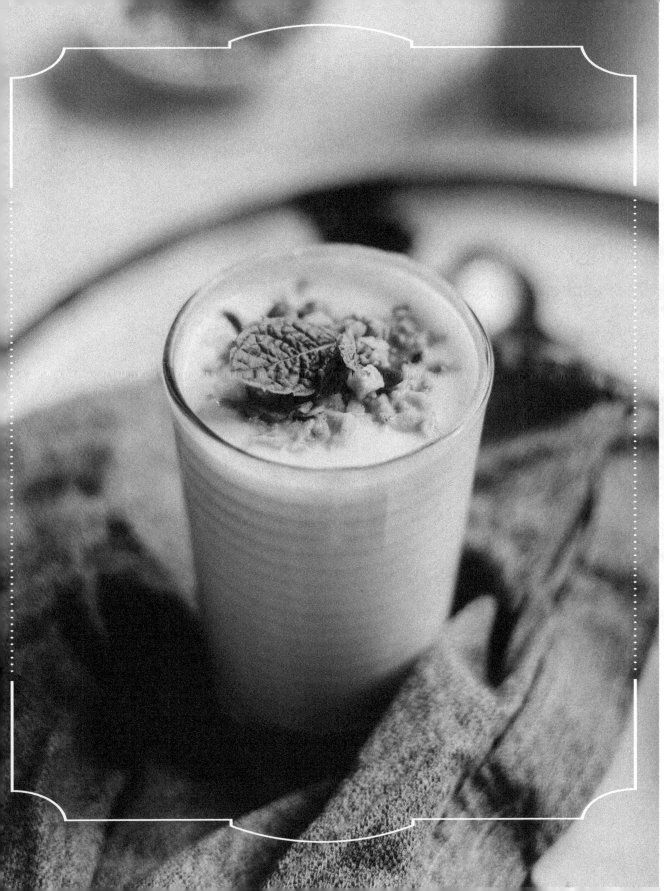

RASPBERRY CHICKEN SALAD

Prep Time: 5 minutes | Cook Time: - minutes | Yield: 1 servings

Ingredients

Raspberry Dressing:

1 cup Yoplait® Fat Free plain yogurt (from 2-lb container)

1/2 cup fresh raspberries

1 tablespoon raspberry or red wine vinegar

2 teaspoons sugar

Salad

6 cups bite-size pieces mixed salad greens (such as Bibb, iceberg, romaine or spinach)

2 cups cut-up cooked chicken breast

1/3 cup thinly sliced celery

1 cup fresh raspberries

Freshly ground pepper, if desired

DIRECTIONS

1. In blender, place dressing ingredients. Cover; blend on high speed about 15 seconds or until smooth.
2. In large bowl, toss salad greens, chicken, celery and 1 cup raspberries. Serve with dressing and pepper.

OVEN BAKED GARLIC AND PARMESAN FRIES

Prep Time: 20 minutes | Cook Time: 40 minutes | Yield: 4 servings

Ingredients

4 large unpeeled russet potatoes, cut into 1/4-inch strips

¼ cup olive oil

3 cloves garlic, minced

½ teaspoon ground dried thyme

¼ teaspoon seasoned salt

½ cup grated Parmesan cheese, divided

¼ cup chopped fresh parsley

¼ cup grated Parmesan cheese

¼ teaspoon seasoned salt

DIRECTIONS

1. Preheat an oven to 425 degrees F (220 degrees C).
2. Place the potatoes in a mixing bowl and drizzle with olive oil. Season with garlic, thyme, and 1/4 teaspoon seasoned salt. Toss until evenly coated. Lift the fries out of the bowl and spread onto a nonstick baking sheet in a single layer. Save the remaining oil in the bowl.
3. Bake in the preheated oven 30 minutes, flipping the fries halfway through baking. Return the fries to the bowl with the olive oil, sprinkle with 1/2 cup Parmesan cheese and parsley. Toss to coat, then spread again onto the baking sheet. Return to the oven, and bake until the Parmesan cheese melts, about 10 minutes. Sprinkle the fries with the remaining 1/4 cup Parmesan cheese and 1/4 teaspoon seasoned salt to serve.

PUMPKIN MUFFINS

Prep Time: 20 minutes | Cook Time: 30 minutes | Yield: 16 muffins

Ingredients

1 cup whole wheat flour

3 tsp. baking powder

2 tsp. ground cinnamon

2 tsp. ground nutmeg

1/4 cup egg substitute

2 Tbsp. Splenda Sugar Blend for Baking

1 cup canned pumpkin

1/2 cup nonfat milk

1/4 cup unsweetened applesauce

1/4 cup raisins or chopped nut

DIRECTIONS

1. Preheat the oven to 400°F.
2. Line 16 muffin-pan cups with paper liners or spray with nonstick cooking spray.
3. In a large bowl, stir together the flour, baking powder, cinnamon, and nutmeg.
4. In a medium bowl, beat the egg substitute with a whisk. Add the Splenda, pumpkin, milk, and applesauce; stir until well blended.
5. Stir the raisins or chopped nuts into the flour mixture until just blended.
6. Fill the muffin-pan cups 2/3 full.
7. Bake 20 to 25 minutes, or until a wooden toothpick inserted in the center comes out clean.
8. Remove the muffins from the pans. Serve warm or at room temperature.

GARLIC LIME CHICKEN WITH OLIVES

Prep Time: 20 minutes | Cook Time: 35 minutes | Yield: 4 servings

Ingredients

1 pound chicken breast halves ; boneless

1 cup onions ; diced

2 cloves garlic ; minced

2 tablespoons lime juice

1 tablespoon molasses

2 teaspoon worcestershire sauce

1 1/2 teaspoon ground cumin

1 teaspoon dried oregano

1/2 teaspoon salt

1/2 teaspoon ground black pepper

1/2 cup greek olives ; pitted and sliced

8 sprigs thyme

2 tablespoons each freshly chopped parsley and basil plus more to garnish

1 teaspoon dried oregano

150 ml red wine

28 oz (820g) crushed tomatoes

2 tablespoons tomato paste

7 oz (200g) Roma tomatoes, halved

1/2 teaspoon red pepper flakes

DIRECTIONS

1. Preheat oven to 400 degrees F.
2. Coat a large roasting pan with cooking spray.
3. In a large bowl, combine chicken, onion, garlic, lime juice, molasses, Worcestershire sauce, cumin, oregano, salt, and black pepper. Toss to coat.
4. Transfer chicken to prepared pan and pour over any remaining marinade. Arrange olives over and around chicken in pan. Roast 30 to 35 minutes, until chicken is cooked through.

PUMPERNICKEL TEA SANDWICHES

Prep Time: 15 minutes | Cook Time: 35 minutes | Yield: 6 servings

Ingredients

6 large hard-cooked eggs, peeled

1/3 cup mayonnaise

1/4 cup minced fresh chives

1/4 cup finely chopped fresh mint

2 teaspoons lemon zest

2 teaspoons Dijon mustard Salt and pepper to taste

1 1/3 cups loosely packed arugula

1 cup very thinly sliced radishes

1 tablespoon lemon juice

1 tablespoon olive oil

14 pumpernickel bread slices

DIRECTIONS

1. Mash eggs with mayonnaise and next 4 ingredients until well blended. Season with salt and pepper to taste. Cover and chill up to 1 day.

2. Toss together arugula, radishes, lemon juice, and olive oil. Season with salt and pepper to taste. Toss to coat.

3. Spread egg salad mixture on 1 side of each bread slice; top 7 slices with arugula mixture. Top with remaining 7 bread slices, egg salad side down. Trim crusts from sandwiches; cut each sandwich into 3 rectangles with a serrated knife

PORK AU POIVRE

Prep Time: 20 minutes | Cook Time: 35 minutes | Yield: 4 servings

Ingredients

1 tablespoon black peppercorns

4 (1/2-inch-thick) rib pork chops (bone in)

1 teaspoon salt

2 tablespoons vegetable oil

1/4 cup medium-dry or cream Sherry

1/3 cup heavy cream

DIRECTIONS

1. Coarsely crush peppercorns by gently pounding once or twice with a heavy skillet. Pat chops dry and sprinkle both sides evenly with salt and peppercorns, pressing to help them adhere.

2. Heat 1 tablespoon oil in a 12-inch heavy skillet over moderate heat until hot but not smoking, then cook 2 chops, turning over once, until browned and just cooked through, 4 to 6 minutes total. Transfer to a plate and wipe out skillet. Cook remaining 2 chops in remaining tablespoon oil in same manner, transferring to plate. (Do not wipe out skillet after second batch.)

3. Add Sherry to skillet and boil, scraping up any brown bits, until reduced by half, about 1 minute. Add cream and any meat juices accumulated on plate, then boil, stirring occasionally, until slightly thickened, about 2 minutes. Season sauce with salt and serve over chops.

GINGER TEA CAKE

Prep Time: 20 minutes | Cook Time: - minutes | Yield: 4 servings

Ingredients

1 tablespoon butter or ghee

Half cup honey

1/4 cup water

1tsp dried ginger powder

1 cup whole-wheat flour

1 tsp garam masala

1 tsp baking powder

1 tsp vanilla extract

1 tsp baking soda

3 eggs

DIRECTIONS

1. Preheat oven to 180C.
2. In an oven-safe bowl, place butter paper or baking sheet.
3. Whisk together - butter/ghee, honey, water, ginger powder, vanilla essence, baking powder and baking soda.
4. Crack eggs on it and whisk again.
5. Add flour in parts, gradually, and keep whisking till it turns into a fine paste. Sprinkle garam masala.
6. Bake and eat.

CHICKEN KEBABS

Prep Time: 20 minutes | Cook Time: 15 minutes | Yield: 6 servings

Ingredients

1 cup plain whole milk Greek yogurt

2 tablespoons olive oil

2 teaspoons paprika

1/2 teaspoon cumin

1/8 teaspoon cinnamon

1 teaspoon crushed red pepper flakes (reduce to 1/2 teaspoon if you don't like heat)

Zest from one lemon

2 tablespoons freshly squeezed lemon juice, from one lemon

1-3/4 teaspoons salt

1/2 teaspoon freshly ground black pepper

5 garlic cloves, minced

2-1/2 pounds boneless skinless chicken thighs, trimmed of any excess fat and cut into large bite-sized pieces

1 large red onion, cut into wedges

Vegetable oil, for greasing the grill

DIRECTIONS

1. In a medium bowl, combine the yogurt, olive oil, paprika, cumin, cinnamon, red pepper flakes, lemon zest, lemon juice, salt, pepper and garlic.

2. Thread the chicken onto metal skewers, folding if the pieces are long and thin, alternating occasionally with the red onions. Be sure not to cram the skewers. (Note: You'll need between 6-8 skewers.) Place the kebabs on a baking sheet lined with aluminum foil. Spoon or brush the marinade all over the meat, coating well. Cover and refrigerate at least eight hours or overnight.

3. Preheat the grill to medium-high heat. To grease the grill, lightly dip a wad of paper towels in vegetable oil and, using tongs, carefully rub over the grates several times until glossy and coated. Grill the chicken kebabs until golden brown and cooked through, turning skewers occasionally, 10 to 15 minutes. Transfer the skewers to a platter and serve.

GRILLED SALAD WITH HERBED VINAIGRETTE

Prep Time: 20 minutes | Cook Time: 15 minutes | Yield: 2 servings

Ingredients

Herbed Vinaigrette

1 tablespoon olive oil

2 teaspoons cider vinegar

1 teaspoon chopped fresh parsley

¼ teaspoon chopped fresh thyme

¼ teaspoon chopped fresh rosemary

⅛ teaspoon salt

1 teaspoon Dash ground pepper

Vegetable Salad

1 medium eggplant, cut crosswise into 1/2-inch-thick slices

1 medium onion, cut into 1/2-inch-thick wedges (see Tip)

2 eaches green and/or red bell peppers, halved, stems, membranes, and seeds removed

6 small 6 large cremini mushrooms, stems removed

3 eaches plum tomatoes, halved lengthwise

3 tablespoons olive oil

1 tablespoon cider vinegar

1 sprig Fresh thyme

DIRECTIONS

1. For vinaigrette, whisk together olive oil, cider vinegar, parsley, thyme, rosemary, salt, and pepper; set aside.
2. For vegetable salad, combine eggplant, onion wedges, bell peppers, mushrooms, and tomatoes in a very large bowl. Add olive oil and cider vinegar. Toss to coat vegetables.
3. Place vegetables on rack of an uncovered grill directly over medium-hot coals. Grill for 3 minutes; turn vegetables. Grill for 3 to 4 minutes more or until vegetables are tender.
4. To serve, cut each pepper half into 3 strips. Arrange vegetables on a platter. Drizzle with reserved vinaigrette. Serve warm or at room temperature. If desired, garnish with fresh thyme.

BANANA CREAM PIE

Prep Time: 10 minutes | Cook Time: - minutes | Yield: 8 servings

Ingredients

1 (3 1/2 ounce) package sugar-free instant banana cream pudding mix

1 1⁄2 cups cold 1% low-fat milk

1 (8 ounce) container Cool Whip Free, thawed and divided

1 large banana, peeled and sliced

1 baked pie shell

DIRECTIONS

1. Mix pudding and milk in a medium bowl.
2. Stir 1 1/2 minutes with a wire whisk.
3. Gently fold 1 cup of Cool Whip Free into pudding mixture.
4. Fold in banana slices.
5. Top with remaining Cool Whip Free.
6. Cover and chill at least 30 minutes.

STRAWBERRY AND TOFU SMOOTHIE

Prep Time: 10 minutes | Cook Time: - minutes | Yield: 2 servings

Ingredients

12 oz tofu

1 cup strawberries (chopped)

1 cup almond milk

2 tablespoons almond butter

1 teaspoon lemon juice

1 teaspoon vanilla extract

½ cup ice cubes

DIRECTIONS

1. Add all of the ingredients to the blender except for the ice cubes. Blend until smooth.
2. Add the ice cubes to the blender and blend until completely smooth.
3. Add desired toppings and serve immediately.

CHILLI BEAN SOUP WITH AVOCADO

Prep Time: 20 minutes | Cook Time: 30 minutes | Yield: 6 servings

Ingredients

1 tbsp oil

1 large onion, chopped

2 cloves garlic, crushed

2 red chillies, finely chopped

1 tsp ground cumin

½ tsp ground cinnamon

2 x 420g tins kidney beans, drained and rinsed

1 x 400g tin chopped tomatoes

1.2L vegetable stock

For the salsa:

1 avocado, peeled and finely chopped

2 tomatoes, finely chopped

4 tbsp fresh coriander,

chopped

half small red onion, finely chopped

half

small red chilli, sliced (optional)

freshly ground black pepper

DIRECTIONS

1. Heat the oil in a large pan, add the onion, garlic and chillies and fry for 2-3 minutes until the onion begins to soften. Add the spices and continue to fry for a further minute.
2. Add the remaining soup ingredients to the pan, bring to the boil, cover and simmer for 20 minutes.
3. Transfer the soup to a food processor or use a stick blender and process until smooth (it may be easier to do this in batches), return to the pan and heat through. Meanwhile, mix together all the ingredients for the salsa.
4. Serve the soup topped with a spoonful of salsa.

SEARED GREENS WITH RED ONION AND VINEGAR

Prep Time: 12 minutes | Cook Time: - minutes | Yield: 4 servings

Ingredients

2 tbsp Vegetable oil

1/2 Red onion ; sliced

1 tsp Mustard seed

1 1/2 lb Red or yellow Swiss chard ; stems removed and tops coarsely chopped

1/4 cup Red wine vinegar

Salt and pepper to taste

DIRECTIONS

1. Heat a large skillet over high heat.
2. Add oil then onion and mustard seeds.
3. Sear onion and mustard seeds, 2 minutes.
4. Add greens and toss with tongs in oil.
5. Sear greens 2 to 3 minutes.
6. Add vinegar and toss with greens. Remove pan from heat and season greens with salt and pepper.

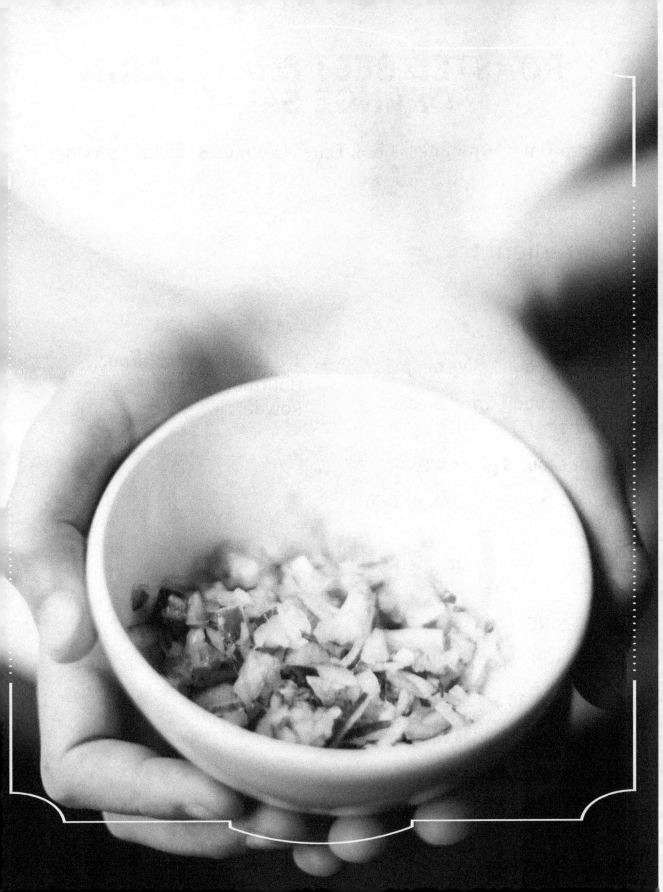

ROASTED BEET & MANDARIN ORANGE SALAD

Prep Time: 15 minutes | Cook Time: 45 minutes | Yield: 4 servings

Ingredients

SALAD

4 small beets

2 tablespoons olive oil

1/2 teaspoon Grind Black Pepper

4 cups mixed greens

1/2 cup sections of mandarin orange, drained

1/4 cup coarsely chopped walnuts, toasted

DRESSING

1 tablespoon olive oil

1/4 cup orange juice

1 tablespoon cider vinegar

1 teaspoon Flat Leaf Parsley

1/4 teaspoon salt

1/8 teaspoon McCormick Gourmet™ Organic Garlic Powder

DIRECTIONS

1. Preheat oven to 375°F. Trim beets, leaving 1 inch of stems and roots; wash. Place beets, 2 teaspoons of the oil and 1/4 teaspoon of the pepper in large resealable plastic bag. Toss to coat beets. Place beets on shallow baking pan

2. Roast 40 to 45 minutes or until fork tender. Cool beets. Peel and cut into 1/2-inch wedges

3. Mix orange juice, remaining 1 tablespoon oil, vinegar, parsley, remaining 1/4 teaspoon pepper, salt and garlic powder in small bowl with wire whisk until well blended

4. To serve, place 1 cup mixed greens on each of 4 plates. Top each with mandarin orange sections and beets. Sprinkle with walnuts and drizzle with dressing

SPAGHETTI WITH SWISS CHARD AND PECORINO

Prep Time: 25 minutes | Cook Time: 45 minutes | Yield: 4 servings

Ingredients

8 oz whole wheat spaghetti (4 servings if you're using one of those spaghetti-measuring discs with holes)

salt, for pasta cooking water (I used fine grind sea salt)

12-16 oz. fresh chard leaves, cut into crosswise strips

1 T finely minced fresh garlic

Optional: pinch of red pepper flakes

1/4 cup extra virgin olive oil

1/4 cup hot pasta cooking water (remove before draining pasta)

1/2 cup coarsely grated Pecorino-Romano cheese (or use any hard grating cheese with a good flavor such as Parmesan or Asiago)

fresh ground black pepper to taste

DIRECTIONS

1. Bring a large pot of water to a boil, adding a generous amount of salt (enough that the water tastes slightly salty.)
2. When water is boiling, add the spaghetti, stir once, reduce heat slightly and boil until the spaghetti is cooked but still slightly chewy or al dente. Consult the spaghetti package for recommended cooking time, but for my Italian whole wheat spaghetti, this took exactly 9 minutes.
3. Grate the Pecorino-Romano or Parmesan cheese on the largest holes of a cheese grater, then coarsely chop with chef's knife, keeping the cheese pieces fairly large.
4. Cut chard leaves into crosswise strips about 1/2 inch wide, cutting out large inner chard stems if needed.
5. Wash chard strips and spin dry or dry with paper towels.
6. In the largest heavy frying pan you have, heat the olive oil over medium heat, add minced garlic (and hot pepper flakes if using) and saute garlic about 1 minute. Be sure not to let the garlic get brown or it can easy turn bitter. It's done when you start to smell garlic.
7. Add chard strips all at once and saute 1-2 minutes, just until chard is wilted down to about half the size it was.
8. Use a measuring cup to remove 1/4 cup hot pasta cooking water and add to chard, then reduce heat to the lowest

possible setting to keep the chard warm.

9. As soon as pasta is cooked but still slightly chewy, drain pasta in a colander placed in the sink, then add hot pasta to the pan with the cooked chard and toss. (I used two large forks to toss the pasta with the chard.)

10. Add about half the grated cheese and toss again.

11. Season to taste with fresh ground black pepper, then divide spaghetti on four individual plates, top each serving with cheese, and serve hot.

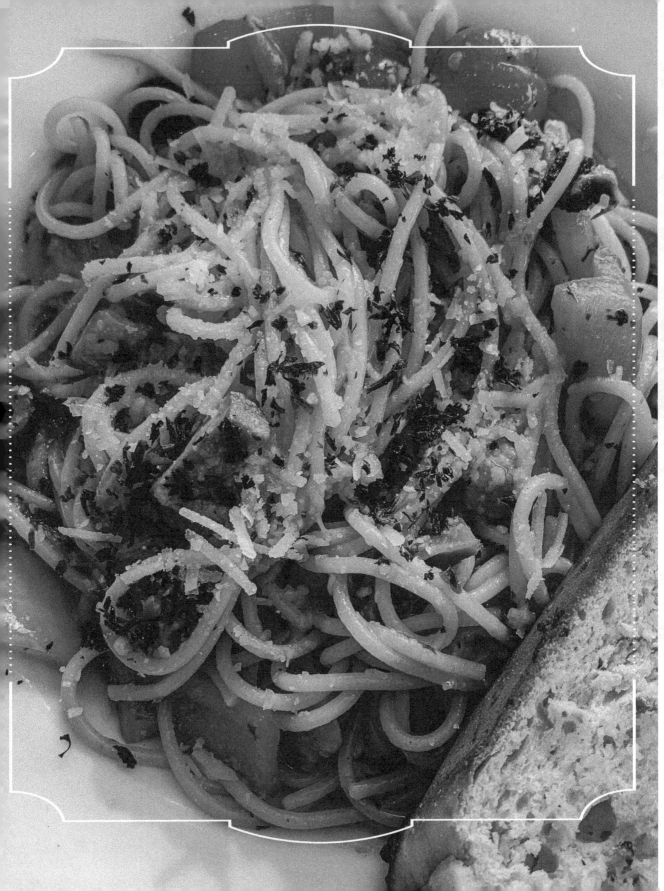

PIMIENTO GREEN BEANS

Prep Time: 5 minutes | Cook Time: 10 minutes | Yield: 10 servings

Ingredients

2 pounds fresh green beans, cut into 2-inch pieces

1 can (14-1/2 ounces) chicken broth

1/2 cup chopped onion

1 jar (2 ounces) chopped pimientos, drained

1/2 teaspoon salt

1/8 to 1/4 teaspoon pepper

1/4 cup shredded Parmesan cheese

DIRECTIONS

1. In a large saucepan, bring beans, broth and onion to a boil. Reduce heat; cover and cook for 10-15 minutes or until crisp-tender. Drain. Stir in pimientos, salt and pepper. Sprinkle with Parmesan cheese.

BLUEBERRY SAUCE

Prep Time: 10 minutes | Cook Time: 10 minutes | Yield: 2 cups

Ingredients

2 cups fresh or frozen blueberries (no need to thaw before use if frozen)

¼ cup water OR apple juice/orange juice, if you want a sweeter sauce

2 tsp. arrowroot powder

1 Tbs. water

DIRECTIONS

1. Place the berries and ¼ cup water (or juice) in a small saucepan over medium heat. Cook for 5-10 minutes, until bubbling. Slightly smash some of the blueberries with the back of a fork.

2. In a small bowl, stir together the arrowroot powder and 1 Tbs. of water. Remove the saucepan of berries from the heat. While stirring constantly, add the arrowroot mixture into the blueberry mixture. Let cool until no longer hot and serve. The sauce with become even thicker when chilled.

3. Store the sauce in the fridge for a few days.

CARROT GREEN APPLE MINT SALAD

Prep Time: 25 minutes | Cook Time: 45 minutes | Yield: 4 servings

Ingredients

1/3 Cup Plain Greek Yogurt

2 Tablespoons Mayonnaise (organic)

1 Tablespoon Lemon Juice

1 Tablespoon Apple Cider Vinegar

1 Teaspoon Honey

1 Pound Carrots peeled and trimmed

1 Granny Smith Apple, cored

2 Tablespoons roughly chopped fresh Mint Leaves

Salt

1/2 Cup Raisins

DIRECTIONS

1. In a small bowl whisk together the thickened yogurt and the mayonnaise, until smooth. Whisk in the lemon juice, vinegar, and honey.

2. Grate first the carrots and then the apples in a food processor. Transfer them to a large bowl and stir to combine. Pour the dressing over the carrot mixture and toss. Add the mint and season with salt.

TOFU AND VEGETABLE STIR-FRY

Prep Time: 35 minutes | Cook Time: 25 minutes | Yield: 4 servings

Ingredients

10 ounces firm tofu, cut into 1/2- to 3/4-inch cubes

1/3 cup lite (low-sodium) teriyaki sauce

1 tablespoon peanut oil

1 teaspoon minced garlic

1 small onion (2 inches in diameter), peeled and diced

1/4 teaspoon black pepper

1/4 cup low-sodium, fat-free chicken broth

1/2 teaspoon lite (low sodium) soy sauce

8 ounces broccoli florets, cut into bite-size pieces

4 ounces fresh white mushrooms, cleaned and quartered

1 small red pepper (about 2–2 1/2 inches in diameter), stemmed, seeds removed, chopped into bite-size pieces

1/2 cup sliced water chestnuts, drained

3 cups cooked brown rice (prepared according to package directions)

DIRECTIONS

1. Place tofu pieces in a small bowl. Pour teriyaki sauce over cubes and stir to coat. Let sit 30 minutes to marinate at room temperature. Meanwhile, prepare vegetables as described above. Heat 1 tablespoon peanut oil over medium-high heat in a wok or large sauté pan. Add garlic, onion, and black pepper and stir-fry about 1 minute. Raise heat to high, and add marinated tofu (and any remaining teriyaki sauce within the bowl), chicken broth, and soy sauce; stir-fry 1 minute. Add broccoli, mushrooms, red pepper, and water chestnuts. Stir-fry 2–3 minutes until desired crispness of vegetables is reached. Serve each portion over 2/3 cup hot, cooked brown rice.

11

50 Mouth-Watering Diabetc Recipes That Taste Like Absolute Heaven

DIABETIC DATE DAINTIES

Ingredients:
1 1/2 tsp. liquid sweetener
1 1/2 tsp. baking powder
1/3 c. dates, chopped
1/4 c. flour
1/2 c. nuts
1 1/2 c. bread crumbs

Directions:
Beat eggs, sweetener and baking powder. Add dates, flour and nuts. Stir in bread crumbs. Chill, then measure by teaspoon on a greased cookie sheet. Bake at 375 degrees for 12 minutes.

SUGAR - FREE CRANBERRY RELISH

Ingredients:
2 c. cranberries
2 apples
1 c. orange juice

Directions:
Grind together the cranberries and apples, using a sweet apple. (May also use blender). Add orange juice, chopped nuts and sweetener to taste. Refrigerate several hours before using.

IT COULD BE A SNICKERS BAR

Ingredients:
12 oz. soft diet ice cream
1 c. diet Cool Whip
1/4 c. chunky peanut butter
1 pkg. sugar-free butterscotch pudding (dry)
3 oz. Grape-Nuts cereal

Directions:
Mix first 4 ingredients in mixer, then stir in cereal. Pour into 8 inch square pan. Cover and freeze. Makes 4 servings.

BAKED CHICKEN FOR ONE

Ingredients:
1 (3 oz.) chicken breast, boned & skinned
2 tbsp. (any brand) bottled diet Italian dressing

Directions:
Marinate chicken in dressing overnight in covered casserole. Bake for one hour at 350 degrees. No additional seasonings are necessary. Will be very tender and juicy.

CHOCOLATE CHIP COOKIES

Ingredients:
1/4 c. margarine
1 tbsp. granulated fructose
1 egg
1 tsp. vanilla extract
3/4 c. flour
1/4 tsp. salt
1/2 c. mini semi-sweet chocolate chips

Directions:
Cream together margarine and fructose , beat in egg, water and vanilla. Combine flour, baking soda and salt in sifter. Sift dry ingredients into creamed mixture, stirring to blend thoroughly. Stir in chocolate chips. Drop by teaspoonsful onto lightly greased cookie sheet about 2 inches apart. Bake at 375 degrees for 8 to 10 minutes. Makes 30 cookies.

BROWNIE TORTE

Ingredients:
1 1/2 c. chilled whipping cream
3 tbsp. Fruit Sweet or to taste
1 tsp. vanilla
1/2 c. pecans, chopped

Directions:
Prepare Fudge Sweet Brownies (see recipe below). Whip cream, Fruit Sweet and vanilla and use as filling and topping for layers of brownies. Low-

Fat Substitute: About 3 cups frozen whipped topping, thawed. Substitute your favorite flavoring for the vanilla, such as 1 tablespoon instant coffee or 1 tablespoon concentrated orange juice.

FROZEN APRICOT MOUSSE

Ingredients:
1 c. apricot apple butter
1/2 c. whipping cream
2 egg whites
2 tbsp. Fruit Sweet

Directions:
Beat egg whites until stiff but not dry. Fold into the apricot apple butter. Whip the cream until stiff, adding the Fruit Sweet. Fold the whipped cream into the apricot mixture. Freeze.

RASPBERRY MOUSSE

Ingredients:
2/3 c. Strawberry Fanciful
1/8 tsp. cream of tartar
2 egg whites
1/2 c. whipping cream

Directions:
Add cream of tartar to egg whites, beat until stiff, but not dry. Fold into Strawberry Fanciful. Fold the whipped cream into the fruit mixture. Chill before serving or freeze for

frozen mousse. For flavor variation try: Strawberry, blueberry, orange pineapple, pineapple berry or peach.

FANCIFUL FREEZE

Ingredients:
4 ripe bananas, peeled
1/2 c. Raspberry Fanciful

Directions:
Wrap bananas in plastic wrap and freeze overnight. Remove from freezer, break into 4 or 5 pieces and let stand at room temperature for about 10 minutes to slightly soften for the processor.   Blend the bananas in a processor or blender until creamy. Add the Raspberry (or other flavor) Fanciful and blend briefly. This can be served immediately, or stored in the freezer. Serves 4.

NO-SUGAR CUSTARD

Ingredients:
6 egg yolks
1/4 c. Fruit Sweet
1/2 c. flour
2 c. milk
1 tsp. vanilla
1 tbsp. butter

Directions:
In a medium bowl, beat egg yolks and Fruit Sweet until thick and pale. While continuing to beat, gradually

sift in flour. Pour into a saucepan and place over low heat on the stove and gradually add milk and vanilla. Cook, stirring constantly, until mixture has thickened to a custard consistency, about 15 minutes. Remove from heat. Melt butter and pour over custard to prevent a skin from forming while it cools. Makes 3 cups.

ORANGE SHERBET (FOR DIABETICS)

Ingredients:
1 c. orange juice
1 tsp. unflavored gelatin (1/3 envelope)
2 tbsp. lemon juice
1 tbsp. grated orange peel nonnutritive sweetener equal to 1/2 cup sugar
1/2 c. nonfat dry milk powder

Directions:
Mix all ingredients together until well blended.

DIABETIC APPLE PIE

Ingredients:
Pastry for 8 inch two crust pie
6 c. sliced tart apples
3/4 tsp. cinnamon or nutmeg
1 (12 oz.) can frozen Seneca apple juice
2 tbsp. cornstarch

Directions:

Heat oven to 425 degrees. Put apples in pastry lined pan. Heat juice, cornstarch and spice (optional). Let it boil until clear. Pour over apples. Cover with top crust. Bake 50 to 60 minutes.

STRAWBERRY DIABETIC JAM

Ingredients:
1 c. berries
3/4 c. sugar-free strawberry pop
1 pkg. strawberry sugar-free Jello
3 packets Equal
Directions:
Mash the berries, add soda pop and cook 1 minute. Remove from heat and stir in Jello until dissolved. Stir in sweetener and pour in jars. Seal and store in refrigerator. Yields about 1 1/4 cups. You may use other fruits such as raspberries, peaches or cherries.

DIABETIC PUNCH

Ingredients:
1-2 liter diet Sprite
1 (46 oz.) can chilled unsweetened pineapple juice
1 pkg. blueberry Kool-Aid with Nutrasweet
Directions:
Chill all ingredients and pour in punch bowl and serve.

NO BAKE DIABETIC FRUIT CAKE

Ingredients:
1 lb. graham crackers, crushed (reserve 3 double crackers)
1/2 lb. margarine
1 lb. marshmallows
Directions:
Melt above and add cracker crumbs. 3/4 c. grated raisins 1 tsp. coconut flavoring 1/2 c. dried apricots 1/2 c. raw cranberries 3/4 c. dates, cut up Add to first mixture and mix well. Pat mixture in 6"x13"x2" pan lined with plastic wrap. Chill.

DIABETIC RAISIN CAKE

Ingredients:
2 c. water
2 c. raisins
Directions:
Cook until water evaporates. Add: 2 eggs 2 tbsp. sweetener 3/4 c. cooking oil 1 tsp. soda 2 c. flour 1 1/2 tsp. cinnamon 1 tsp. vanilla Mix well. Pour into 8"x8" greased pan, bake at 350 degrees for 2 minutes. Makes 20 servings. 1 fruit, 2 fat, 185 calories.

DIABETIC SPONGE CAKE

Ingredients:
7 eggs
1/2 c. fruit juice, orange
3 tbsp. Sweet 'n Low or any sugar substitute
2 tbsp. lemon juice
3/4 tsp. cream of tartar
1 1/2 c. sifted cake flour
1/4 tsp. salt
substitute
2 tbsp. lemon juice
3/4 tsp. cream of tartar
1 1/2 c. sifted cake flour
1/4 tsp. salt

Directions:
Separate eggs. Beat egg whites with salt until foamy. Add cream of tartar and continue beating until stiff. In another bowl, combine rest of ingredients and mix well. Fold in beaten egg whites. Bake in greased and floured bundt pan at 350 degrees for 40 minutes or longer; test with toothpick. Serve with no sugar jelly (all fruit) and Cool Whip.

MARY TYLER MOORE'S ALMOND MERINGUE COOKIES (DIABETIC)

Ingredients:
4 egg whites
8 tsp. powdered skim milk
1 tsp. vanilla extract
1 tsp. almond extract
1 tsp. liquid artificial sweetner
Cinnamon to taste

Directions:
Beat egg whites until stiff. Add skim milk powder. Mix well. Add extracts and sugar substitute. Drop cookies by spoonfuls onto cookie sheet. Bake at 275 degrees for 45 minutes. Remove from cookie sheet and dust with cinnamon. Yields 2 to 2 1/2 dozen. One cookie equals 32 calories.

DIABETIC BREAD PUDDING

Ingredients:
1 slice white bread, cut in cubes
2 or 3 tbsp. raisins
1 c. skim milk

1 egg, well beaten
2 pkgs. artificial sweetener
1 tsp. vanilla
Directions:
Beat egg, milk, vanilla and sweetener together. Spray two (2) cup microwave dish with non-sticking vegetable spray. Arrange bread cubes and raisins in dish. Pour milk mixture over bread to moisten each cube. Sprinkle dash of nutmeg over top and microwave on high for five (5) minutes or until knife inserted in center comes out clean. Be careful not to overcook.

DIABETIC PEANUT BUTTER COOKIES

Ingredients:
1/2 c. peanut butter
1 tbsp. low calorie oleo
2 1/2 tsp. liquid sweetener
2 eggs
1 c. flour
1/4 tsp. soda
1/2 c. skimmed milk
Directions:
Beat first 4 ingredients well. Add eggs and beat again, then add milk and flour. Blend well. Drop by spoon on cookie sheet that is greased well. Bake at 375 degrees for 12 minutes.

DIABETIC BROWNIES

Ingredients:
2 c. graham cracker crumbs (approximately 24 crackers)
1/2 c. chopped walnuts
3 oz. semi-sweet chocolate
1 1/2 tsp. Sweet-N-Low (6 packs)
1/4 tsp. salt
1 c. skim milk
Directions:
Heat oven to 350 degrees. Place all ingredients in bowl; blend well. Bake in greased 8x8x2 pan for 30 minutes. Cut in 2-inch squares while warm.

DIABETIC JELLY

Ingredients:
1 c. unsweetened juice (any kind)
1/4 tsp. lemon juice
2 tbsp. sugar substitute
1 tbsp. plain gelatin
1 tbsp. cornstarch
Directions:
Mix lemon juice, sugar substitute, gelatin and cornstarch. Add fruit juice and stir well to mix. Boil hard for 3 minutes, stirring constantly. Makes 1 small jar. Store in refrigerator.

ANNE'S DIABETIC CHOCOLATE SYRUP

Ingredients:
1/3 c. dry cocoa
1 1/4 c. cold water
1/4 tsp. salt
2 tsp. vanilla
3 tsp. liquid sweetner
Directions:
Combine all ingredients; bring to full boil. Simmer 20 minutes.

DIABETIC CINNAMON COOKIES

Ingredients:
1 slice bread, crumbled
1/4 tsp. cinnamon
1/4 tsp. vanilla
1 egg, beaten
1 tsp. sweetener
Directions:
Mix all ingredients together, drop on cookie sheet, bake at 350 degrees for about 10 - 15 min or until lightly brown.

DIABETIC EASTER FUDGE

Ingredients:
1 sq. unsweetened chocolate
1/4 c. evaporated milk
1/2 tsp. vanilla
1 tsp. artificial liquid sweetener
1 pkg. vanilla or chocolate sweetened pudding powder
8 tsp. finely chopped nuts
Directions:
Mix all ingredients together and bring to a boil over med. heat, stirring constantly. When mixture begins to thicken , quickly pour into pan or dish to cool and set. May be refrigerated to hasten cooling.

SPICED TEA (DIABETIC)

Ingredients:
1 c. instant tea with NutraSweet
2 pkg. Kool aid
Sunshine Punch with NutraSweet
1 tsp. cinnamon
1 tsp. cloves
Directions:
Add desired portion to cup of hot water.

DIABETIC CRANBERRY AND ORANGE SALAD

Ingredients:
1 lb. fresh cranberries
1 med. orange, do not peel
1 med. apple, do not peel
1 lg. celery stalk

Directions:
Grind the above ingredients together. 1 (3 oz.) box orange sugar free Jello 2 tbsp. Equal sweetener Dissolve Jello in 3/4 cup boiling water; add 3/4 cup cold water. Add ground fruit, celery, pineapple, sweetener. Chill.

DIABETIC GLORIFIED RICE

Ingredients:
1/2 c. rice, uncooked (not instant)
1 (20 oz.) crushed pineapple, in own juice
1 (3 oz.) pkg. sugar-free fruit flavored gelatin
Boiling water
Pineapple juice, drained from can
Maraschino cherries
Heavy cream

Directions:
Cook rice according to package directions. Drain, set aside. Drain pineapple, reserving 1 cup juice. Dissolve gelatin in 1 cup boiling water. Add juice. Stir in well drained rice, the cooked rice will absorb the color and flavor of the gelatin. Mix well and chill until thickened but not quite set. Add drained pineapple and cherries, if desired. Fold in cream that has been whipped. Chill. Makes about 8 servings.

DIABETIC CREAM CHEESE SALAD

Ingredients:
1 (3 oz.) env. sugar free Jello (lime)
1 c. crushed pineapple in own juice
3 oz. lite cream cheese, room temperature
1/2 c. evaporated skim milk, chilled
1 med. orange, do not peel
1 med. apple, do not peel
1 lg. celery stalk

Directions:
Mix Jello per package directions. Drain juice from pineapple and add water to make 1/2 cup liquid. Add juice to Jello mixture and chill until syrupy. Beat the evaporated skim milk, making sure that the bowl, beaters and milk are well chilled. Set whipped milk aside. Beat the cream cheese into Jello. Fold in the whipped milk and drained pineapple

and chill in mold or glass dish. Makes 9 ½-cup servings.

EASY SUGAR-FREE DESSERT

Ingredients:
1 (6 oz.) pkg. sugar-free Jello
2 c. hot water
1/2 pkg. Crystal Light lemonade mix
2 c. water
3 c. Cool Whip
1 angle food cake
Directions:
Dissolve Jello in hot water. Add lemonade mix and water. Chill until slightly thickened, beat until frothy and fold in Cool Whip. Fold in cake broken in pieces. Put into 9 x 13 inch pan and chill.

CREAM PUFFS

Ingredients:
½ Margarine
1 c. boliling water
1 c. flour
½ tsp salt
4 eggs
Directions:
Melt margarine in 1 cup boiling water. Sift flour and salt together. Add to boiling liquid all at once and stir until mixture leaves side of pan in compact ball. Cool 1 minute. Put in mixing bowl and add eggs -

one at a time, beating well after each addition. Drop by rounded teaspoon onto ungreased cookie sheet. Bake at 450 degrees for 10 minutes and then at 400 degrees for about 25 minutes. Cool and fill with favorite filling. Suggested filling: 1 tub Cool Whip, stir in 1/2 package instant vanilla pudding.

SUGARLESS APPLE PIE

Ingredients:
1 (12 oz.) can frozen apple juice concentrate, thawed
3 tbsp. cornstarch
1/4 tsp. salt
1 tsp. cinnamon
1/2 tsp. nutmeg
5-6 apples, peeled, cored and sliced
Directions:
Mix all ingredients, bring to a boil. Pour into crust-lined pie plate. Top with remaining crust. Bake at 425 degrees about 45 minutes until crust is golden and apples are tender.

SMAKEROON COOKIES

Ingredients:
3 egg whites
1/2 tsp. cream of tartar
2 tsp. sugar substitute
1/4 tsp. almond flavoring
3 c. Rice Krispies

1/4 c. shredded coconut

Directions:

Beat egg whites until foamy, add cream of tartar and continue beating until stiff but not dry. Add sugar substitute and flavoring. Beat until blended. Fold in cereal and coconut and drop by teaspoonfuls onto lightly greased cookie sheet. Bake at 350 degrees for 12-15 minutes or until lightly browned. 1 serving = 1 fruit exchange (3 cookies). Yields 24 cookies.

CHOCOLATE SAUCE

Ingredients:

1 tbsp. butter
2 tbsp. cocoa
1 tbsp. cornstarch
1 c. skim milk
2 tsp. sugar substitute
1/8 tsp. salt

Directions:

Melt butter. Combine cocoa, cornstarch and salt; blend with melted butter until smooth. Add milk and sugar substitute and cook over moderate heat, stirring constantly until slightly thickened, remove from heat. Stir in vanilla. Set pan in ice water and stir until completely cold. (Sauce thickens as it cools.) One serving - (1 tablespoon) free exchange.

DIETETIC PASTA SALAD

Ingredients:

Corkscrew pasta
4 fresh mushrooms, sliced
1 cucumber, sliced
Kraft reduced calorie zesty Italian dressing
1 onion, sliced
1 tomato, diced
1 green pepper, chopped

Directions:

Cook and rinse pasta in cold water. Mix with remaining ingredients and marinate in dressing. Chill and serve.

SUGAR FREE APPLE PIE

Ingredients:

4 c. sliced, pared apples (preferably yellow delicious)
1/2 c. unsweetened apple juice concentrate (do not dilute)
1 1/2 tsp. cornstarch or tapioca
1 1/2 tsp. cinnamon or apple pie spice

Directions:

Mix thickener, concentrate, and spices. Pour over apple slices to coat well. Pour into crust-lined pie plate. Top with remaining crust. Bake at 425 degrees about 45 minutes until crust is golden and apples are tender. 8 servings each 220 calories. Exchanges = 1 1/2 fruit, 1 bread, 1/2 fat each serving.

DIABETIC CHEESE CAKE

Ingredients:
2/3 c. cottage cheese
1/3 c. cold water
1/2 tsp. vanilla
1/2 c. blueberries
1/3 c. hot water
1/3 c. powdered milk and 3 pkgs. Equal
1 tsp. lemon juice
1 env. unflavored gelatin

Directions:
Soften gelatin in cold water, then add hot water. Blend until smooth. Add rest of ingredients and blend again until smooth. Stir in blueberries. Chill until firm.

DIABETIC PUMPKIN PIE

Ingredients:
1 sm. pkg. sugar-free vanilla pudding
1 1/2 c. milk (whole or nonfat)
1 c. canned pumpkin
1/4 tsp. cinnamon
1/4 tsp. nutmeg
Artificial sweetener to equal 1 tsp. sugar
1 baked 8-inch pie crust

Directions:
Place pudding mix in a saucepan. Gradually add milk. Cook and stir over medium heat until mixture comes to a boil. Remove from heat and add pumpkin, spices and sweetener;

mix well. Pour into baked crust. Chill until firm, about 3 hours.

DIABETIC WHIPPED CREAM

Ingredients:
1/3 c. instant nonfat dry milk
1/3 c. ice water
1/2 tsp. liquid sweetener

Directions:
Chill small glass bowl and beaters. Combine ingredients and whip on high speed with mixer until consistency of whipped cream. Makes about 10 servings of 2 tablespoons.

STRAWBERRY PIE (NO SUGAR)

Ingredients:
1 baked pie shell
1 qt. strawberries
3 tbsp. cornstarch
1 (8 oz.) pkg. cream cheese
1 c. apple juice, unsweetened

Directions:
Slice berries, simmer 1 cup in 2/3 cups apple juice 3 minutes. Mix cornstarch with 1/3 cup apple juice, stir in berries. Stir constantly 1 minute until thick. Spread softened cheese over pie crust,

put berries on cheese, pour cooked berries on top. Garnish with whipped cream and a few berries. Chill 3 to 4 hours.

POPSICLES

Ingredients:
1 (4 serving size) env. sugar-free gelatin
1 (2 qt.) env. sugar-free artificially sweetened powdered drink mix (Kool-Aid)

Directions:
In a 2 quart mixing pitcher, dissolve gelatin in 1 cup hot water. Add drink powder; stir, then add 7 cups cold water. Stir. Pour into popsicle cups with handles; freeze. Flavor Suggestions: Raspberry Lemonade Orange Orange Grape Gelatin: Triple berry Lime Hawaiian pineapple Strawberry Raspberry These pops will not melt easily because of the absence of sugar. 1 (2 ounce) popsicle = 2 to 3 calories. 5 to 6 may be eaten per day and is considered a "free" food.

POLISH SAUSAGE STEW

Ingredients:
1 can cream of celery soup
1/4 c. brown sugar
27 oz. can sauerkraut, drained
1 1/2 lb. polish sausage, cut in 2 inch pieces

4 med. potatoes, pared and cubed
1 c. chopped onion
4 oz. shredded Monterey Jack cheese

Directions:
Cook sausage,potatoes, and onion until done. Mix soup, sugar & sauerkraut, cook until blended. Mix with other ingredients and top with cheese.

KRAUTRUNZA

Ingredients:
1 link (approximately 1/4 lb.) German sausage
1 lb. ground beef
1 sm. head cabbage
1 med. onion
Salt and pepper
Yeast dough

Directions:
Brown meats and add other ingredients, cook until tender. Serve

GERMAN SAUERKRAUT

Ingredients:
1 can Bavarian sauerkraut, partially drained
1 apple, cored and sliced
1 onion, chopped
2 or 3 slices bacon

Directions:
Mix together and cook until all is tender.

PATCHLINGS

Ingredients:
5 c. flour
1 egg
1 tbsp. shortening
1 c. milk

Directions:
Mix all ingredients together,
drop on cookie sheet, and bake at 350
degrees for about 10 min.

WALNUT DREAMS

Ingredients:
¼ lb margarine
1 ½ c. + 1 tbsp brown sugar
1 ½ c. chopped walnuts
2 eggs (beaten)
1 ½ tsp baking powder
1 tsp vanilla
½ c. coconut

Directions:
Mix all ingredients together and blend
thoroughly. Drop on cookie sheet , bake
at 325 degrees until lightly brown.

MOM'S WIENER SOUP

Ingredients:
4 wieners
1 onion
1 qt. milk
1 1/2 tsp. salt
4 tbsp. butter
2 tbsp. flour
2 c. cooked, diced potatoes
1/4 tsp. pepper

Directions:
Brown potatoes, wieners and onions
in 2tbsp butter. Mix milk, salt, pepper,
flour and other 2 tbsp butter together,
stir constantly until mixture boils and
becomes smooth. Then mix everything
together in a soup pan or pot, cook
until everything is hot, then serve.

IOCOA EGG PANCAKES

Ingredients:
8 eggs, whip hard
1 tsp. salt
2 1/2 c. milk or water
1 c. flour

Directions:
Mix all ingredients and pour onto grill.
Cook on each side until lightly brown.

TUNA SUPREME

Ingredients:
1 sm. can tuna, water-packed
3 hard boiled eggs, diced
1 c. American cheese, diced
2 tbsp. each chopped sweet pickles, mince onion, chopped celery and cut-up stuffed olives
1/2 c. mayonnaise or Miracle Whip

Directions:
Mix all ingredients and serve on bread or lettuce leaf.

DIABETIC SPICY MEATBALLS

Ingredients:
1 lb. lean ground beef
1/2 c. chili sauce
2 tsp. prepared horseradish
1/2 c. minced onion
2 tsp. Worcestershire sauce
1/2 tsp. salt
2 tbsp. corn oil

Directions:
Mix all ingredients well, roll into balls, and brown in corn oil. Drain on paper towels.

PORK CHOPS & STUFFING

Ingredients:
5 pork chops
1 box croutons, prepared to box directions, as stuffing
1/4 c. water

Directions:
Brown pork chops, make sure cooked well. Serve with stuffing.

BANANA BREAD

Ingredients:
2 c. all purpose flour
1 tsp. baking soda
1 tsp. baking powder
1 1/2 tsp. pumpkin pie spice
2 ripe bananas (mashed)
6 oz. can frozen orange juice
2 eggs
1 c. raisins
Nuts (optional)

Directions:
Sift all dry ingredients together and set aside. In a separate bowl mix all wet ingredients and mashed bananas. Mix wet and dry ingredients together and mix well, then fold in, nuts and raisins. Pour in a greased and floured loaf pan unless using a non-stick pan. Bake at 350 - 375 degrees for 30-45 minutes or when knife comes out clean.

BUTTERMILK SHERBET

Ingredients:
2 c. buttermilk
Sugar substitute equal to 1/2 c. sugar
1 egg white
1 1/2 tsp. vanilla
1/2 to 1 cup crushed pineapple
Directions:
Combine and blend well all ingredients
except pineapple. Pour into container.
Add pineapple. Freeze. Stir
occasionally until firm.

CPSIA information can be obtained
at www.ICGtesting.com
Printed in the USA
BVHW010019240621
610312BV00014B/98

9 781801 920636